Coping with Obsessive Compulsive Disorder

Professor Kevin Gournay is Emeritus Professor at the Institute of Psychiatry (Kings College, University of London). In his clinical work he treats OCD, phobias and other anxiety disorders, and post-traumatic stress disorder. He has worked in areas of general medicine including pain management, cardiovascular disorders and multiple sclerosis, and has researched on CBT, violence, suicide, schizophrenia, medication, phobias, body image disorders, epidemiology, health economics and primary care. He is the author of 300 books, chapters and papers. He is President and founding patron of the charity No Panic, and is a frequent contributor to the media. In 2004 he was elected as 'Psychiatric Nurse of the Year' by the American Psychiatric Nurses Association. He lives in Hertfordshire and has four children.

Rachel Piper is a wife, mother, employee and artist with a very vivid imagination, who is fully aware of the incapacitating nature of OCD. In trying to overcome her own OCD and clinical depression, she has learned to channel her imagination in a positive way by capturing the beauty of the world through her camera. She strongly believes that an obsessive mind can also bring gifts, such as creativity. Rachel was first diagnosed with OCD in 1989, but diagnosis took several years. For this reason she eventually discovered a determination to be more open, and she acknowledges all those who suffer from OCD and the families who support them. In sharing her experiences she hopes to help others find the courage and determination to confront their own fears.

Professor Paul Rogers qualified as a psychiatric nurse in 1989. He later trained in behavioural/cognitive behavioural therapy and worked as a clinical nurse specialist in CBT at the Caswell Clinic Medium Secure Unit in South Wales, specializing in people traditionally considered not amenable to psychological therapy. For his PhD he studied the association between command hallucinations and violence, and was then awarded a post-doctoral research fellowship to study suicidal thinking in prisoners. In 2004 he was appointed Chair of Forensic Nursing at the University of Glamorgan. Throughout his academic training he has continued to see clients weekly for CBT (specializing in OCD and PTSD). He has published over 100 professional and peer review papers, research reviews and book chapters.

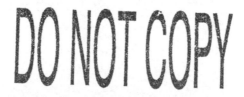

Overcoming Common Problems Series

Selected titles

A full list of titles is available from Sheldon Press,
36 Causton Street, London SW1P 4ST and on our website at
www.sheldonpress.co.uk

101 Questions to Ask Your Doctor
Dr Tom Smith

Asperger Syndrome in Adults
Dr Ruth Searle

The Assertiveness Handbook
Mary Hartley

Assertiveness: Step by step
Dr Windy Dryden and Daniel Constantinou

Backache: What you need to know
Dr David Delvin

Birth Over 35
Sheila Kitzinger

Body Language: What you need to know
David Cohen

Bulimia, Binge-eating and their Treatment
Professor J. Hubert Lacey, Dr Bryony Bamford
and Amy Brown

The Cancer Survivor's Handbook
Dr Terry Priestman

The Chronic Pain Diet Book
Neville Shone

Cider Vinegar
Margaret Hills

Coeliac Disease: What you need to know
Alex Gazzola

Confidence Works
Gladeana McMahon

Coping Successfully with Pain
Neville Shone

Coping Successfully with Prostate Cancer
Dr Tom Smith

Coping Successfully with Psoriasis
Christine Craggs-Hinton

Coping Successfully with Ulcerative Colitis
Peter Cartwright

Coping Successfully with Varicose Veins
Christine Craggs-Hinton

Coping Successfully with Your Hiatus Hernia
Dr Tom Smith

Coping Successfully with Your Irritable Bowel
Rosemary Nicol

Coping When Your Child Has Cerebral Palsy
Jill Eckersley

Coping with Asthma in Adults
Mark Greener

Coping with Birth Trauma and Postnatal Depression
Lucy Jolin

Coping with Bowel Cancer
Dr Tom Smith

Coping with Bronchitis and Emphysema
Dr Tom Smith

Coping with Candida
Shirley Trickett

Coping with Chemotherapy
Dr Terry Priestman

Coping with Chronic Fatigue
Trudie Chalder

Coping with Coeliac Disease
Karen Brody

Coping with Diverticulitis
Peter Cartwright

Coping with Drug Problems in the Family
Lucy Jolin

Coping with Dyspraxia
Jill Eckersley

Coping with Early-onset Dementia
Jill Eckersley

Coping with Eating Disorders and Body Image
Christine Craggs-Hinton

Coping with Envy
Dr Windy Dryden

Coping with Epilepsy in Children and Young People
Susan Elliot-Wright

Coping with Gout
Christine Craggs-Hinton

Coping with Hay Fever
Christine Craggs-Hinton

Coping with Headaches and Migraine
Alison Frith

Coping with Heartburn and Reflux
Dr Tom Smith

Coping with Kidney Disease
Dr Tom Smith

Overcoming Common Problems Series

Overcoming Common Problems Series

Overcoming Common Problems

Coping with Obsessive Compulsive Disorder

PROFESSOR KEVIN GOURNAY
RACHEL PIPER
PROFESSOR PAUL ROGERS

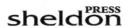

First published in Great Britain in 2012

Sheldon Press
36 Causton Street
London SW1P 4ST
www.sheldonpress.co.uk

British Library Cataloguing-in-Publication Data
A catalogue record for this book is available from the British Library

ISBN 978-1-84709-157-4
eBook ISBN 978-1-84709-239-7

Typeset by Caroline Waldron, Wirral, Cheshire
Printed in Great Britain by Ashford Colour Press
Subsequently digitally printed in Great Britain

Produced on paper from sustainable forests

Dedications

PROFESSOR KEVIN GOURNAY

For Sam – with memories of sorbet in the American Colony

RACHEL PIPER

For David

PROFESSOR PAUL ROGERS

For Allison, Clara and Hannah – thank you

PUBLISHER'S DEDICATION

For Soulla Thalis, who first suggested the idea of this book

Contents

Acknowledgements

We here acknowledge some of the people who have influenced us most in our respective careers and who have inspired us to write this book.

First and foremost, we must mention Professor Isaac Marks, who taught Professors Gournay and Rogers at the Maudsley Hospital. Professor Marks, as well as being one of the world's leading authorities on the nature and treatment of fears and phobias, was at the forefront of the development of treatments for OCD some 40 years ago. The experience gained training in his unit has been absolutely invaluable and many of the basic lessons learned then are still being applied today.

Over the years, Professor Gournay has been inspired by the privilege of working with a number of leading authorities on OCD. In particular, his collaboration with Dr David Veale in the early part of the 1990s was both fruitful and enjoyable in their study of a very close relative of OCD, body dysmorphic disorder (BDD). This included in-depth interviews with and assessments of some 50 individuals, as a result of which they conducted a pilot study of treatment and developed a model for cognitive behavioural treatment. Dr Veale has gone on to pursue this work further and has become a leading authority on OCD and BDD. This work has left an enduring impression, and the lesson learned is that complex cases demand patience, thought and the need to continually refer to the evidence available. People with OCD and BDD can sometimes be very difficult to treat and often do not respond to the first methods that one employs. If one does not achieve a suitable response to treatment, it is essential to reflect on the reasons why and to set new objectives with new methods, or a different mixture of methods, and then reassess outcomes. In the case of the most difficult-to-treat people, this process may go on for some time.

Professor Gournay is indebted to all those involved with No Panic, the self-help charity with which he has been involved for the past 20 years, in particular, the founder and chief executive the late Colin Hammond, who sadly died in November 2011. With his wife Marion, Colin led the work of this charity since it was founded. The UK's largest self-help organization for anxiety disorders, No Panic has won numerous national awards, including the Queen's Award for Voluntary Service (in 2004) and the Charity of the Year Award (in 2003) and has a primary focus on people suffering from phobias and panic. Of the more than 70,000 calls a year received by No Panic, there are many from people with OCD, because of the acute anxiety engendered by the condition.

Professor Paul Rogers has been practising as a CBT therapist for nearly 20 years and has had the privilege of working with many close colleagues who have happily given advice during this time. He would like to thank the senior staff at the Caswell Clinic in Bridgend who originally seconded him to undertake the 18-month nurse therapy training at Professor Isaac Mark's unit at the Maudsley Hospital.

He is grateful to Mrs Ruth Davis and Professor Maggie Kirk at the University of Glamorgan for their counsel and support, and Dr Peter Jenkins, consultant psychiatrist in Cardiff, who has always provided excellent advice and mentorship on a range of issues. He also thanks Professor Gournay for being such a good friend and close colleague.

Most importantly, Professor Rogers is indebted to all the clients he has seen with OCD (and BDD) over the last 20 years for letting him into their private worlds. So often, clients are ashamed or embarrassed about their obsessive thought or compulsive behaviours, and he never fails to be impressed by clients' honesty, sincerity and determination in overcoming their problems.

Rachel Piper would like to thank her family, in particular, David, Naomi and Rebecca, for always loving her and helping her to learn; living with somebody else's OCD is not always easy. She would also like to express her appreciation of the special people for whom she has great admiration: Professor Gournay, together with Professor Rogers and all those who work towards helping people overcome this incapacitating disorder.

Introduction

Why a self-help book on OCD?

It is true that there are already a number of very good self-help books on OCD. However, some of these books do not lend themselves particularly to a UK readership, as they are written with a USA audience in mind. Second, some of the self-help books that we have seen, good as they are, appear to us to be daunting to many potential readers because of their length and, at times, the excessive technical emphasis, which may be off-putting to many people.

We have set out to produce a book that is relatively short, easy to read and, at the same time, contains advice based on evidence from the highest-quality research studies so far carried out. We offer advice based on solid scientific evidence. In doing so, we make no apologies for concentrating on the psychological treatment approach with the best supportive evidence – that is, cognitive behavioural therapy (CBT). However, at the same time we accept that the cognitive behavioural approach does not have all the answers. We know, from our shared experience and from our reading of numerous scientific studies, that some people show little or no benefits from CBT, that some people respond well to medication alone, and that, sadly, a small proportion show no response to either approach. As our knowledge advances, it is becoming clear that OCD is not a single condition, but rather an umbrella term that covers a number of related conditions. In this book we attempt to describe the main forms of OCD and provide advice on how to deal with its various manifestations.

Although in the very recent past the UK government has made attempts to improve the training of health professionals so that they are better able to deliver treatment for conditions like OCD via the Improving Access to Psychological Therapies (IAPT) programme, it is still a sad fact that, for the foreseeable future, most people will never receive the evidence-based treatments that they need, delivered by an appropriately trained professional, because of the shortage of such suitable professionals. Thus, as with other anxiety states, self-help in its many forms will continue to be a necessity. However, this picture is not as gloomy as it sounds. We know that self-help can be very effective and, indeed, our experience from working with self-help organizations tells us that many people with anxiety states appear to obtain excellent results when using methods based on self-help. We also know that self-help materials, such as this book, may be used very effectively as an aid to professional treatment.

NICE guidelines

Throughout this book, we refer to the 2005 NICE guidelines for OCD and BDD. NICE (National Institute for Health and Clinical Excellence) is an independent organization set up by the government to be responsible for providing national guidance on promoting good health and preventing ill health. NICE has several functions, one of them being the production of clinical guidelines.

These clinical guidelines are based on the best available evidence at that time. NICE guidance assists health professionals in their work by setting out the treatment approaches to clinical conditions, which are supported by evidence from high-quality research studies. Such guidance is now recognized as the very best way to proceed, and if anyone recommends a treatment that is not based on NICE guidance, they need to be able to justify very clearly why they have done so. It is now accepted that not following NICE guidance may be deemed negligent.

NICE guidelines are reviewed at approximately five-yearly intervals, and the NICE website contains a huge amount of information concerning each and every guideline. The website is relatively easy to navigate and you will see that guidelines come in several versions, including a very helpful one for the general public, written in plain English. These versions are by no means 'dumbed down'; a great deal of work goes into translating technical language into a form that may be understood by the intelligent lay person. These versions usually consist of 20 to 30 pages. Interested members of the general public may, of course, download the more technical information, which is provided for health professionals.

Structure of the book

Essentially, the book comes in two parts. The first provides information about OCD in its various forms, including case histories based on real people. We know that case studies help readers identify with their own problems, and over the years we have often been told that such descriptions help people to feel greatly comforted. Often for the very first time, people with OCD realize that they are by no means alone and that their problems are not unique; and, perhaps more importantly (particularly with OCD), that they have no reason to feel shame or guilt because of their condition. We also describe the treatments available, so that people with OCD who read this book have the necessary knowledge when dealing with a health care system that may place obstacles on the pathway towards receiving appropriate care and treatment. This part of the book concludes with Rachel's account of the way in which OCD has affected her, the benefits of professional treatments and the strategies she has adopted in order to lead a productive and fulfilling life. Rachel also describes 'Oscar', a character she has developed as part of a novel self-help strategy.

The second half of the book is devoted to a self-help programme, set out in a very practical way. The book concludes with a list of resources, books, organizations and references for further reading.

Part 1
OCD: The facts

1

Defining OCD

Professionals define OCD principally through the two classification systems used in the English-speaking world: the *Diagnostic and Statistical Manual*, published by the American Psychiatric Association (APA) and currently in its fourth edition (DSM-IV), and the International Classification of Diseases, published by the World Health Organization, currently in version 10. Nevertheless, OCD is quite difficult to define because it can present in a number of ways. The principal manifestations of OCD are in the form of:

- Obsessions, which are also commonly known as obsessional thoughts and/or ruminations. These terms mean exactly the same thing.
- Compulsions, which are also known as compulsive actions or rituals. These terms mean exactly the same thing.
- A combination of obsessions (ruminations) and compulsions (rituals).

Obsessions (ruminations)

The NICE guidance, published in 2005, defines an obsession as 'an unwanted or intrusive thought, image or urge that repeatedly enters the person's mind'.

If you ask people with obsessions, they will tell you that they realize that these intrusive thoughts or images are irrational, and are, as we shall demonstrate in some of the case examples in this book, alien to their nature. Obsessions, by definition, cause considerable distress and anxiety and can severely affect day-to-day functioning.

In the vernacular we use the word 'obsession' to describe something someone thinks about all of the time, and it is not uncommon to hear phrases such as an obsession with football, or an obsession with Elvis Presley. Such 'obsessions' usually give the person a great deal of pleasure and they have at some point decided that they would rather occupy their mind with the focus of the obsession, rather than other life matters. Such obsessions are not the focus of this book. Anyone who has known someone with obsessional thoughts will recognize the enormous distress that these thoughts cause. Another defining characteristic of obsessions is that people will do, or try to do, everything that they can in order to try and resist them coming into their mind; the severity of such resistance can be very extreme.

Madeline

Madeline had always been a devout Roman Catholic; she attended Mass every Sunday, went to confession twice a month and was always present on important days in the church calendar – for example, during Holy Week. Madeline describes herself as someone with a social conscience, who has always been guided by a strong Christian philosophy. Madeline's obsession arose following a period of prolonged stress, when she began to worry that she might 'blurt out' something that she did not mean to say while in church. This developed into Madeline thinking of the names of Christ, the Virgin Mary and the disciples, coupled with gross obscenities. Whenever she entered a church, she was overwhelmed by the fear that she might blurt out phrases involving a combination of holy names and gross obscenities. Very quickly, these combinations of names and obscenities came into her mind at various, random times during the day, and she soon became depressed because she thought she had sinned by having such thoughts.

We will later on describe how such patterns of thinking and fears are overcome. It is worth noting now, however, that Madeline responded to treatment and she was greatly comforted when she was told by her therapist that such thoughts are quite common in people with obsessions.

Compulsions

Compulsions are different. They are defined in the NICE guidance as 'repetitive behaviours or mental acts that the person feels driven to perform'.

Some compulsions are often very clearly observable by others – for example, excessive washing and cleaning, or the repetitive checking of locks, switches and taps. Sometimes, however, they are only experienced by the person themselves – for example, needing to repeat to oneself a certain phrase a set number of times.

Examples of common compulsions include repetitive behaviours associated with ideas of being unclean or contaminated, or the checking of light switches, door locks or gas taps, with the fear that not checking these items will lead to some harm befalling the person or their family.

As you can see, the definitions of obsessions and compulsions have some overlap and there is often a link between thoughts and actions, although not necessarily always.

Richard

Richard, while successful in his education and career, describes himself as 'always a worrier'. He recalls, during his school days, becoming very concerned about catching illnesses from others. This worry often caused him to lose sleep. He also developed the compulsive washing of his hands to prevent being infected with viruses and bacteria. Over time Richard began to carry antibacterial wipes wherever he went and became concerned about eating foods that might cause him 'a stomach upset'. This led him to check the contents of his fridge and throw out foods that he thought were close to their sell-by date. Richard began to avoid social situations for fear of catching infection and stopped eating out in restaurants. Just before he attended for an assessment of his problem he was using two packets of antibacterial wipes each day, and several bars of soap a week, and his hands were red and inflamed because of excessive hand-washing. He had also just thrown out the entire contents of his fridge because he found a yogurt that was one day from reaching its sell-by date. His contamination fears were causing problems with his marriage. His wife complained that Richard's avoidance, excessive cleaning and the restrictions he imposed on their everyday life had begun to overwhelm all other aspects of their life together. She also mentioned that their conversations were increasingly dominated by Richard's fears.

In the second part of this book we will describe how compulsions and fears, such as Richard's, can be overcome. Indeed, we have to say at this point that Richard's problems are much more common in the general population than one would think.

Shelley

Shelley was 18 and had been accepted by Cambridge University to undertake a BSc in physics. She had always been a high achiever and was committed to her studies and future academic career. At the time of referral she was taking a gap year and working as a volunteer at her local university. She got on very well with her parents and siblings and had plenty of friends. Over the previous 18 months she had gradually begun developing fears that something 'awful' was going to happen to her family (including her grandparents). To counteract the anxiety that such thoughts caused, she developed a number of 'rituals', which at first she did discreetly but over time became increasingly obvious due to her need to ritualize more and more.

She had three main rituals. The first was checking that the taps in the upstairs bathroom were off and not dripping. She would turn the taps on and off seven times, and on the seventh time tighten the tap as hard as she could before trying to leave the bathroom. The second was turning her bedroom light switch on and off 14 times and then on the fourteenth time repeatedly telling herself, 'It's off, it's off,' before trying to exit the room. The third was dragging her foot across the areas in the house where two different types of carpets met. However, she would often think that her foot 'jumped up' or didn't maintain perfect contact with the carpet during the dragging ritual, so she would have to repeat this until she was satisfied. This could, at worst, take up to an hour to complete before Shelley was satisfied.

Obsessions and compulsions combined

Perhaps the most common presentation of OCD is the combination of obsessions and compulsions. In the cases of Richard and Shelley, above, those around them could observe their compulsive behaviour and, at first sight, one could say that this was the central problem. Richard's widespread compulsive behaviour, principally focused on hand-washing, checking and avoidance behaviours, was underpinned by his fears of being infected, while Shelley's fears were focused on 'some unknown harm' befalling her family.

We will demonstrate in the second part of the book how to deal with problems such as Richard's and Shelley's, and in such cases one needs to focus on both the obsessions, and the compulsions that result. Turning back to the case of Madeline, none of her friends or family observed any changes in her behaviour apart from noticing that, as her obsessions worsened (the nature of these obsessions she kept very much to herself), she appeared more withdrawn and depressed. Such obsessions often lead to behavioural manifestations, such as avoidance, as happened with Madeline; before she came for treatment, she was avoiding attending some, though not all, of the church services that were a normal part of her religious observance, and this, therefore, fed back into her fears that she was a 'bad' Christian.

How common is OCD?

At one time OCD was seen as a rare disorder but it is now commonly accepted that between 1 and 2 per cent of the population have the condition to a degree that warrants treatment. The National Institute for Mental Health in the USA has collected a vast amount of evidence concerning the prevalence of OCD and information can be found on their website.[1] For the academically minded, this website provides a long list of publications describing various studies carried out to estimate prevalence.

An issue that is of great concern when one considers that there are perhaps up to one million people with OCD in the UK is the availability of treatment. Even with significant advances in the development of treatments and the training of health professionals, it seems clear that only a tiny proportion of those with OCD are likely to receive effective treatment. Apart from the scarcity of treatment resources within the NHS, people may not come forward as they are ashamed of their problem, particularly if their fears centre around harming others or entertaining thoughts that other people might find disagreeable. An individual may take the decision to endure their condition in silence because they do not see it as a solvable problem; rather, it is something they have to live with. In addition, there is the issue of approaching a professional for help within the wider context of the stigma attached to mental health problems.

Children and adolescents with OCD

OCD often begins in childhood, and it is estimated that more than 50 per cent of adults affected remember their OCD beginning during their childhood years. OCD is more common in younger boys, but by the time adolescence is reached there are equal numbers of boys and girls with the disorder. The most common forms of OCD in children concern rituals of symmetry, counting, and having things in a particular order. Sometimes they are referred to as safety and security rituals, because unless things are done in a particular way or a particular number of times, the child may fear that something dreadful will happen to them or to others. Children may simply feel very uncomfortable if things are not done in a certain way or a certain number of times.

It is important to realize that some obsessive behaviour occurs in many children, but this is not necessarily a sign that they are developing OCD. Simple superstitions, such as stepping on a crack in the pavement, are common and some children engage in harmless rituals before they go to sleep, to make them feel safe. Quite simply, most children grow out of this developmental phase. Children have a need to seek reassurance from their parents and there is, of course, a parental responsibility to provide this reassurance appropriately. However, children with OCD may develop patterns of seeking reassurance that quickly get out of hand. It is now accepted that if one can recognize OCD at an early stage, interventions can be very beneficial and prevent the problem developing to a more substantial form in later life. We advise that children showing OCD-like behaviour should be assessed, by a paediatrician or a child and adolescent mental health service professional, because this may be part of another condition, such as autistic spectrum disorder.

The line between normal and abnormal

Before going any further, we must make the point that the vast majority of us will recognize some traits common to OCD in ourselves. For example, most of us will remember, as children, some magical or superstitious thinking or ritualistic behaviour. Comfort rituals with children are a part of normal development. Many people are uneasy about walking under a ladder, or will touch wood, throw spilled salt over their shoulder, salute a magpie, and so on. One needs to remember that superstitions are so common that some hotels do not have a room 13 and some do not have a thirteenth floor!

More subtly, some individuals have a sense of responsibility that could be described as slightly disproportionate. Although not so severe that this could be deemed a problem, some people may more readily identify the responsibility they have for their actions and be concerned lest they make errors. Such individuals often worry about their work excessively and may continue to worry after they leave work and go home. On reflection, anyone might wish, of course, that a surgeon carrying out an operation should have these characteristics, because such a surgeon might check, somewhat obsessively, to ensure that no surgical instruments are left in the patient's body after an operation. Similarly, an accountant with a meticulous approach to financial matters is someone in whom we place great reliance and trust. Some people with OCD are, like Madeline described above, guided by religious principles, and they become disproportionately concerned with matters of right and wrong. However, to a lesser extent, this may simply be a characteristic of someone who could be described in their community as a person of the highest moral and ethical standards, someone who might doggedly fight for a good cause. Perhaps the best way of defining OCD as a clinical problem, rather than as an exaggeration of normal personality traits, is to have evidence that the problem upsets or interferes with normal day-to-day activities.

2

Categories of obsessions and compulsions

Obsessions (ruminations)

Below we list of some of the common categories of obsessions. As stated earlier, obsessions are thoughts, images or urges that repeatedly enter one's mind and generally cause distress. This distress may take the form of anxiety, guilt, shame, embarrassment, or any combination of feelings which upset the sufferer. Obsessions also cannot be easily dismissed.

Aggressive obsessions

Aggressive obsessions may take many forms. People commonly worry about harming other people, particularly those who are vulnerable – for example, babies and small children, or the elderly. Often, the obsession involves someone who is much loved. The aggressive acts commonly described involve horrendous levels of violence. Sometimes these are accompanied by mental images. The person will often say that they fear that their aggressive act will take place on impulse, or even that they may wake up in the middle of the night, carry out the aggressive act and then return to bed and forget it. They may worry about somehow causing injury or death to another by failing to make safe the gas or electricity supply. They are often afraid of holding certain objects (such as sharp knives) for fear that somehow they may use them against a family member. A common fear in London is that the person will push someone in front of an oncoming tube train on the underground.

> #### Ian
> Ian was a 47-year-old who had presented with very long-standing obsessive compulsive disorder, which – as is common – had never been revealed to anyone. Because of the shame that he felt, Ian had never approached his GP. However, matters came to a head when Ian went into

a police station to confess that he had knocked someone off a bicycle – or at least, he thought he had done so. Ian had been on a business trip and had driven to a destination some 150 miles away from his home. The journey back involved a number of narrow country lanes, and on one of these lanes Ian recalled passing a man on a bicycle. He was thinking over work problems at the time, so he wasn't concentrating 100 per cent on the road ahead.

A mile or two down the road, he began to think that he may have 'nudged' the man from his bicycle, and he therefore turned his car around and conducted an increasingly frantic search of the location and the hedgerows around where he thought an accident might have occurred. By the time he reached home after abandoning the search, he was in a state of very high anxiety, and this anxiety continued unabated until he went to bed. He then could not sleep, and had to get up to check the news on the TV and internet, to no avail. He even phoned the Accident and Emergency departments in the county he was driving in, to try to ascertain if anyone had been brought in who had been knocked off a bike. At 3 a.m., after having no luck in finding out whether he had caused harm, he went to the local police station to 'confess his crime'.

The local police where the incident had taken place conducted a search but, predictably, found no trace of the cyclist. Ian later told his therapist that all the time he was actually 99.99 per cent sure that there had been no accident, but the anxiety that his uncertainty caused became overwhelming. Eventually he told the police officers about the nature of his fear, and there followed a very embarrassing and anxious period when he thought he might be prosecuted for wasting police time, but the police eventually decided to take no further action.

At assessment it became clear that Ian's life had been punctuated by a number of incidents where he felt that he may have been responsible for a wide range of adverse events, including knocking down pedestrians while driving his car, causing his neighbours to be poisoned by putting protective paint on his fence, or knocking over ladders on which workmen had been standing. He also entertained ideas that he may have got up in the night and gone out to commit a murder or rape. If he was staying alone in a hotel in a particular location, he would scan the papers the next day, listen to the radio and watch the TV for reports of such crimes. If such a crime had been committed in the vicinity, Ian would spend days, or sometimes weeks, in a state of high anxiety because he 'might' have got up in the middle of the night and committed the crime.

The episode with the cyclist that brought Ian to his therapist's attention proved to be positive insofar as it availed him of assessment and treatment. In due course, with quite prolonged cognitive behavioural therapy, Ian – although he is not completely recovered – reports now that his fears are less intense and prolonged, and not so upsetting to his day-to-day activities.

Sexual obsessions

These obsessions often involve thoughts, images, or a combination of thoughts and images, which disgust the individual involved and often lead to profound feelings of guilt and shame. People may report being concerned that they may have previously unknown sexual preferences towards children, or in heterosexuals, towards people of the same gender. There is often the preoccupation that these thoughts will lead to inappropriate sexual behaviour, such as exposing one's genitals in public or impulsively touching someone in a sexual way in the workplace. Consequently, people can develop a range of day-to-day avoidances, which gradually build up and start to affect a person's everyday functioning. For example, one man was worried that he would need to use a public urinal and while doing so might act inappropriately. He began to venture out only to places that were increasingly nearer and nearer to his home, for fear that when out and about he would need to use the toilet, and if nearby he would be able to get back home in time to do so.

Contamination obsessions

Contamination obsessions come in many forms. While a preoccupation with germs and dirt are common, people can become excessively concerned with chemicals, cleaning agents, nuclear material and asbestos. Contamination obsessions often follow world events – for example, following the Chernobyl disaster, people sought treatment, reporting their avoidance of Scotland and the east coast of England because of fears that they may be contaminated by radiation drifting over to the UK. Similarly, following the massive publicity concerning HIV and AIDS some 20 years ago, many people became preoccupied by fears associated with this, reporting their avoidance of, for example, an innocent red mark in a public situation, with the thought that the red mark may be dried blood shed by someone with AIDS. At the same time, the person with the obsession usually realized that even if the innocent red mark was blood, infection with HIV was impossible. In addition, some people reported avoiding walking on beaches or in long grass, for fear that they might step on a 'used' syringe and needle that might be lying hidden and therefore unseen.

Symmetrical obsessions

Many of us have a tidy desk and like things to be 'just so', or have a 'tidy' house. Indeed, there is the well-known saying, 'Everything in its place and a place for everything.' However, symmetrical obsessions, or the need to have objects, thoughts or behaviours ordered in a particular way, go much further. These obsessions are quite common and, as can be imagined, usually lead to behaviours that will result in order being restored. In the case of these obsessions, the person involved will be preoccupied by the need to have order in all they see and all they do, and if such order does not prevail they will become distressed. People with symmetrical obsessions can often provide no logical reason why they need such order to exist – other than to say that a lack of it leads them to become upset. One man was obsessed that all the grass in his lawn must be exactly the same length, and resorted to cutting his lawn using a ruler and very sharp kitchen scissors. Suffice to say, this was an eight-hour ordeal every time it needed to be done. His wife would often suggest that they replaced the grass with pebbles as a means of trying to find a way that would help her husband cope.

Religious obsessions

Religious obsessions come in various forms. As in the case of Madeline, they may involve thoughts that horrify, such as an obscene image coupled with Christ's name. They may take the form of a disproportionate concern with one's moral, ethical and religious code – for example, a Catholic who would normally go to confession every three months might start to feel the need to confess the most minor of transgressions, and therefore to visit the priest weekly, or in some cases that we have seen, daily. In order to understand these obsessions properly, one needs to be aware of the context – thus, what might be 'normal' for one religion or denomination may be 'abnormal' for another.

Hoarding obsessions

Hoarding obsessions involve concerns about throwing things away, or in some way discarding objects that may later prove to be useful. Such obsessions are usually linked with hoarding behaviours. One woman who was referred by her GP was obsessed that she may need a receipt to return items she had bought, some time in the future. She developed a compulsion to store all receipts, but also had to photocopy them, and take a photo of each receipt, in case she lost one. In addition, she had a ledger where she recorded all the salient (and not-so-salient) information for each receipt (what was bought, where, time of purchase, state of goods at time of purchase, any immediate concerns with the item, and so on). She would then store the two sets of receipts, the ledger and the photos in four different places in her home, as she feared that she may be burgled or have a house fire, so losing or causing damage to her receipts/photos/ledger; she believed that the chance of losing all four sources of information would be reduced if she kept them separate.

Bodily obsessions

Many obsessions involve contamination fears. However, the most prominent form of body obsession is body dysmorphic disorder (BDD). Body dysmorphic disorder was previously known as dysmorphophobia, and can also be referred to as body dysmorphia or dysmorphic syndrome – these names all describe the same condition. A person with BDD is excessively concerned about, and preoccupied by, a perceived defect in their physical features or body image.

BDD is diagnosed in those who are extremely self-critical of their image or physique. Often there will be no obvious disfigurement or defect, or if there is a blemish, it will be so small that it is hardly noticeable. The most common areas of the body that those with BDD will feel critical about are the face: the hair, the skin, and the nose. People with BDD will either excessively 'mirror check' – where they have to check their appearance so that it is as 'perfect' as they can get it before being able to leave the mirror – or they can be completely mirror-avoidant (including catching glimpses of themselves in shop windows). Many resort to excessively seeking reassurance from their family or partners about their appearance (and perceived defect), sometimes to the eventual detriment of these relationships; such reassurance-seeking can become frequent, prolonged and associated with high levels of distress.

Dave

Dave attended for CBT when he was signed off sick from work as an on-site engineer for a large manufacturing company. He described a life-long history of shyness and some degree of social anxiety (for example, he always felt anxious when around people in case they negatively evaluated him for some reason). Since the age of 14 he had gradually become preoccupied with his facial appearance, thinking that he was ugly. It was at this age that he reported last being able to look at his reflection with both eyes open, as he had developed a habit of keeping his right eye shut as he preferred the image from his left eye.

As time went on, he also gradually developed fears about going bald, and while he was showing some very slight signs of thinning on top, it was not obviously noticeable. To counteract his fear of going bald he tried every possible product on the market that claimed success in reversing or slowing baldness (including those available on the internet), all to no effect. He had visited numerous doctors seeking an opinion on how to stop going bald, often with the same response – that there was nothing to worry about. In addition, he had stopped washing that part of his hair for fear that the friction caused by shampooing the area may cause more hair loss, and had not washed the crown of his head for over six months. After bathing, he would count the hairs in the bath and if there were more than one or two he would get extremely panicky. Dave frequently asked his parents for reassurance, which gradually, over the months, wore his father down, so that he refused to discuss the subject or have it discussed in his presence. His mother continued to reassure him, though.

Dave rarely left the house for fear of bumping into people that he knew, in case they noticed his hair, and had become virtually housebound. He would only venture out, for a 15-minute walk, once it was dark, as he was less worried about coming across people in the darkness, and if he did they wouldn't be able to see his hair. Not surprisingly, therefore, he had become quite depressed during this time that he had shut himself away and isolated himself from friends and the social activities he used to enjoy.

Miscellaneous obsessions

Although we have, above, covered many of the common obsessions, numerous other obsessions are reported. People may be preoccupied by almost anything one can imagine – for example, fear of losing possessions, making mistakes, blurting things out, with not being able to get enough sleep that night, or generally losing control and doing something embarrassing. Sometimes people become obsessed with their memory. We all suffer memory lapses and, of course, these lapses tend to increase as we get older. Some people become particularly concerned about things they cannot remember, and naturally the more one tries to remember something, the more difficult it becomes to retrieve that particular memory. We all know that we will find our keys and spectacles the moment we stop looking.

Memory fears may lead the person involved to become preoccupied with 'losing their mind', or a fear that they are developing Alzheimer's disease, and so on. One woman, aged 84, had slowly developed a fear that she was losing her memory for people's names. Consequently, she did everything she could to try and prove to herself that she could remember people's names. She watched the BBC news every morning, followed by GMTV and any chat shows later in the day, as all these programmes would invariably have guests being interviewed. She would then try and remember all their names. To make sure, she also had to write their names out on a piece of paper, which had to be checked out on the internet by her 87-year-old husband. At its worst, she would stay awake all night trying to remember someone's name, and had in the past called her daughter 200 miles away, at 3 a.m., asking for help with a name.

In addition, people can become preoccupied by certain numbers and certain superstitions, and although to some extent superstitious behaviour may be seen as normal, particularly in some cultures, for example where certain numbers may be deemed 'lucky', it may develop to become a major preoccupation. There have been cases of people who become so preoccupied by particular numbers that they can only converse in sentences containing a certain number of words. They spend huge amounts of time thinking up appropriate sentences, with the correct number of words. Similarly, people may become preoccupied by particular letters, or numbers of letters.

Compulsions (rituals)

As the previous section shows, obsessions can concern virtually any topic, and obsessions often lead to compulsions. We describe below some of the compulsions commonly seen. This could be a very long list! However, we will confine ourselves to the most common manifestations of compulsions.

As stated earlier, compulsions are repetitive behaviours or mental acts that the person feels driven to perform. They often have the aim of reducing anxiety and/or distress and the associated fears of 'harm' occurring. It is possible for compulsions to overwhelm a person's life.

Cleaning compulsions

Cleaning compulsions usually involve household cleaning, and may be confined to one's own house, where the focus of responsibility lies. However, some cleaning rituals are connected with contamination obsessions and may involve taking cleaning materials to public places – for example, lavatories, restaurants, or other people's homes. Sometimes cleaning has a specific purpose, perhaps to remove dirt or germs. In other cases the cleaning sets out to remove 'contamination' in general. When asked, people often report that they are not quite sure what contamination means, but they will, at the same time, say that they know when they feel uncomfortable because something is non-specifically 'contaminated'. This contamination may lead to feelings of disgust or revulsion.

Washing obsessions

Washing obsessions commonly involve hand-washing. This may be repeated many times, and in the worst cases can take several hours before the person is satisfied that their hands are clean. Hand-washing may involve the use of soap, or chemicals such as alcohol, and be accompanied by excessive scrubbing – for example, with a nail brush. It is not uncommon to see people whose skin is inflamed, cracked or bleeding. Washing obsessions may include the obsessive brushing of teeth, or the cleaning of anal or genital areas, and may involve the use of chemicals and rituals taking place over a number of hours. One woman was so worried and obsessed that she would 'catch a germ' in her vagina and thereafter be unable to conceive and give birth that she would compulsively wash herself up to eight times a day with diluted bleach, in total using a bottle of bleach per day during her washing rituals.

Checking

One can think of many items around the house that can be associated with safety. Gas taps, windows, electric switches, door and window locks, and water taps, may all become the subject of checking. A person may check that all the knives are locked away in the correct drawer (or attic!) and all accounted for (the person may be afraid that they may use a knife to injure a family member when being out of control in some way). A more recent form of checking now concerns emails, mobile phone texts and social networking sites. Some people become overly preoccupied by the fear that they may have missed something important, such as an urgent message. However, drawing the line between normal and abnormal in this 'new' area can be very difficult, as many 'normal' people seem to spend hours checking emails and texts, and on social networking sites.

Checking may involve ensuring over and over that one has not made a mistake – for example, the obsessive reading of something that one has written, and checking to see that one has in fact put a letter in an envelope, or a cheque with a particular bill. Sometimes people check to make sure that they have not written something that would cause embarrassment. It is not uncommon for people to wonder if they may have written a confession to a particular crime and somehow forgotten that they have posted this confession to the authorities.

Repeating and counting

Most 'normal' people may repeat an activity until they feel comfortable that this has been carried out correctly. Thus, although it is understandable that one might want to re-read a letter or an email to check it is correct, re-reading or checking something a specific number of times may become a substantial problem. People with OCD may need to repeat a wide range of daily activities a certain number of times; these activities might include leaving the house and coming in through the front door, dressing, tying up shoelaces, combing one's hair. The need to repeat things a specific number of times may be associated with 'lucky' and 'unlucky' numbers. The problem worsens when the person becomes unsure whether they have counted correctly, and they then need to start the whole sequence again, often meaning that they become 'incredibly slow' on completing some tasks.

Ordering and symmetry

Although many of us like to have things arranged in a particular way, and might be uncomfortable if we see a crooked picture in our living room, ordering and symmetry can become more of a problem for some people. People may spend literally all day arranging things in a particular order. Sometimes this is because not having things in a particular order leads to a general feeling of being uncomfortable, or of being constantly distracted by the thing that is not in order. In other cases, people may be concerned that if things are not put in a particular order, some dire consequence will follow – for example, the death of a loved relative.

Hoarding

One needs to be able to draw the line between collecting and hoarding. We all know people who are avid collectors of stamps, medals, vinyl records, and such like. They generally enjoy what they do, and even if others cannot 'see the fascination' of, say, collecting stamps, one can understand that this particular hobby may take a great amount of time. However, in cases of compulsive hoarding, people hoard materials that have no particular use – for example, newspapers or documents that have no relevance (often just in case they may be needed at some time in the future). Sometimes people hoard for fear of inadvertently throwing away something useful. People's houses can be completely taken over by all manner of hoarded materials. Where the items hoarded are foodstuffs, this may become a source of hazard.

Bodily compulsions

As noted above, body dysmorphic disorder (BDD) involves a preoccupation with bodily parts, and people may endlessly check their body for signs of imperfection. BDD is discussed in more detail below. Bodily compulsions, however, can take other forms. People may mutilate themselves by endlessly picking at skin, for example, or pulling out hair, in a repetitive way. This latter condition is known as trichotillomania, and is often associated with other forms of obsessions and compulsions, although it can occur on its own.

Trichotillomania

This is a condition often neglected in mental health literature. The name comes from the Greek and means 'hair-pulling madness'. Typically, hairs are pulled in a systematic and 'habitual' or compulsive manner, usually from the scalp, eyebrows or eyelashes, although hairs may be pulled from any part of the body, including nasal and pubic hair. Trichotillomania is associated with feelings of unattractiveness, shame and low self-esteem, and problems with interpersonal relationships. Often people will swallow the pulled hairs, which can cause physical complications (for example, abdominal pain, anaemia, nausea and vomiting, bowel obstruction or perforation). Hair-pulling often occurs at times of stress, and is associated with tension either prior to the act or resisting the urge to hair-pull. While hair-pulling, some people report gratification or pleasure.

Trichotillomania is currently categorized as an 'impulse control disorder' in the fourth edition of the *Diagnostic and Statistical Manual* (DSM-IV), although some authoritative writers have argued that trichotillomania falls within the spectrum of obsessive compulsive disorders. There are some subtle differences that help differentiate between trichotillomania and OCD. In OCD the repetitive behaviours are in response to an obsession, or to rules that are rigidly applied; in trichotillomania hair-pulling is usually a purposeful behaviour carried out in the presence of tension. Further, a consideration of a diagnosis of BDD should be considered where the hair-pulling behaviour is primarily concerned with beliefs about appearance.[2]

Sue

Sue was a 36-year-old travel representative who was referred for CBT assessment by her GP. She complained of an inability to resist the urge to pull out her hair at times of distress. This had resulted in noticeable bald patches on her scalp. The problem had started 18 years earlier when, during late adolescence, she began pulling hairs from her scalp and eyebrows in an effort to ensure that her appearance was satisfactory. She subsequently noticed an increase in hair-pulling every time she became anxious or tense. She described being unable to stop pulling her hair.

During hair-pulling episodes she reported that she was 'wholly engrossed' in the activity, and paid great attention to feeling for 'loose' hairs, which she would twirl around her fingers before giving the hair a short, sharp tug to remove it. Once removed, the hair would be placed between the thumb and forefinger of each hand and examined visually. After this the hair was placed between her teeth and rolled between her lips using her tongue. When she experienced a new urge, the old hair was removed from her mouth and placed in the bin.

Each episode lasted between 20 to 30 minutes, during which some 10 to 15 hairs were removed from her head. On average there were three hair-pulling episodes each day. During each episode Sue reported that she felt a sense of 'satisfaction', and when she had finished hair-pulling she described a sense of 'relief'. At times of increased stress, either from work circumstances or life events, the frequency of episodes increased to six or seven each day. She had tried a number of times to 'give up' hair-pulling, but had found that it was impossible to do so as she sometimes did it without noticing, similar to a 'habit'. She also found it hard to cope with the tension and stress that resisting the urge caused her.

Hair pulling caused Sue significant problems. She attempted to conceal her bald patches by wearing a hat or headscarf, by using thickening shampoo and conditioners, and by blow-drying her hair over them. When possible, she would avoid social events, such as parties. She reported feeling ashamed about her behaviour and thought that if people found out about it they would ridicule her. On the occasions where others had noticed her hair loss, she would explain it as a result of a medical condition (alopecia). She had considered buying a wig to conceal her hair loss but was put off by the cost. She also avoided having any sexual relationships for fear of her hair loss being noticed. She very much wanted to develop close relationships with men, but kept 'putting it off' until such a time as her hair had returned to normal. Unfortunately, it never did. Sue's experiences show how severe an episode of trichotillomania can be, not just in terms of the effect on the person's psychological health (self-esteem, anxiety and mood) but of how her behaviour began to affect her relationships and social life.

Miscellaneous compulsions

As with obsessions, an almost infinite number of compulsions can be performed. People may make endless lists, beyond these lists having any useful purpose. People may feel compelled to confess their perceived shortcomings to others, or to ask endless questions. Sometimes people repeat stories that they have already told in a compulsive fashion. Although many of us may tell the same old tale, obsessive telling is different insofar as it involves the need to ensure that all correct information was transmitted. Other people engage in compulsive bodily activities, such as staring, foot-tapping, touching one's head, and so on.

Increasingly, over the last 20 years, we are seeing more people who have OCD related to the obsession of not being able to get a good night's sleep and the worry that their work performance the next day will be 'awful', resulting in some form of work-related ridicule. Invariably, people with these obsessions develop a range of compulsions (and avoidances) that over time add up to an increasingly stressful series of behaviours. These can include having to exercise at the gym nightly, taking certain herbal medications that claim to help with sleep, having a bath at a set time every night, with the customary 'hot milky drink' thereafter. Usually, people with this condition will have set rules and 'procedures' that they must follow (being in bed by a certain time, saying prayers in a certain order, the house being 'just right' so they can relax when going to bed). Some will require the windows to be shut (to block out noise), while others may need them wide open (to allow air to circulate). One woman was so obsessed about being awoken by birdsong or bird noises that, in order to try and dissuade the birds from landing near her house, she completely cleared her rear and front gardens of all shrubs and plants and concreted over the entire space. In addition she had compact discs hanging by string all over both gardens to scare off birds, and installed special spiky protrusions on her roof and guttering to stop them landing on the house.

Eating disorders

Sometimes eating becomes a compulsion, with the need to eat in a certain way, to chew each mouthful a certain number of times, or to eat food in a particular order, at a certain speed (fast or slow). Other examples include having to cut up food, irrespective of whether it is necessary (for example, scrambled eggs, spaghetti); having to prepare food in a certain way, and then eat it in a certain way (slicing a muffin or bagel and placing it upside down, or inside out); mixing strange foods together, or only being able to eat foods if they are in certain combinations (having to eat jam with chicken); eating foods that are lighter in colour first, then darker ones later; eating foods by the order that their first letter appears in the alphabet (and reverse) (chicken, then peas, then potatoes); having 'safe' and 'not-so-safe' foods; placing food in the cupboard by some order that relates to the way it will be selected to be eaten; not allowing food items to touch each other on the plate, and so on.

According to the DSM-IV, there are two main types of eating disorders: anorexia nervosa and bulimia nervosa. People with anorexia have an extreme fear of gaining weight or being 'fat', which in turn leads them to severely restrict their food intake. They struggle to see their bodies in a realistic way, often demonstrating a distorted self-image where they view themselves as overweight even though they are significantly underweight. One main symptom of anorexia is an inability to maintain normal body weight (defined as 85 per cent of a healthy weight, based on an individual's height and age). Unfortunately, people with anorexia also base their self-esteem and self-worth on their perception of their bodies, which is almost always critical, harsh and devaluing.

People with bulimia are also very critical of their body and base their self-worth on this negative perception. This often leads to restrictive eating, and consequent overwhelming hunger, especially late in the day and at night. When hunger becomes unbearable or stress levels are high, bulimic individuals 'binge eat', and in an attempt to ward off weight gain due to this bingeing, engage in purging behaviours, such as self-induced vomiting, laxative abuse, or unhealthy exercising. Ironically, this pattern often leads to weight gain, leaving people with bulimia near or above their healthy weight.

OCD characteristics can be found in people with eating disorders. OCD might lead the person to count calories methodically, exercise an excessive and exact amount, at a specific time every day, to cut up food in a certain order and in specific shapes, to need to have everything perfect (which includes weight and body symmetry), and so on. Because the person is compelled to follow these rituals through, they find it very difficult to just stop them without professional help.

A major difference, however, is the degree of 'insight' or awareness they have. The person with OCD will usually be able to recognize that their obsessions and compulsions are illogical, but still feel compelled to do them. Often, the person with an eating disorder will not be able to see this – for example, someone with anorexia nervosa will truly believe that they are excessively fat and therefore will not view their compulsive behaviours as out of the ordinary. As such, it is extremely important that people with eating disorders have access to and receive proper professional help (including in-patient admissions if necessary), in order to ensure that their weight loss or any OCD-like behaviours (such as vomiting) do not pose a significant risk to their physical health and integrity.

3

Conditions that co-exist or overlap with OCD

Body dysmorphic disorder (BDD)

Body dysmorphic disorder (BDD) is a relatively new term. It was coined by the American Psychiatric Association in 1994 to describe people who have a preoccupation (obsession) with an imagined defect in their appearance. It is also applied when people do have a slight physical anomaly, and become disproportionately preoccupied with it. Some people attempt to change their perceived body imperfection by camouflaging it with make-up, or even having plastic surgery. Generally, however, such strategies do not help and, in fact, often make the problem worse.

For many years this condition was thought to be very rare, but it is in fact quite common. People with BDD are very reluctant to come forward for treatment, and often when they do they have great trouble providing comprehensive information about their difficulties, usually because of a great sense of embarrassment or shame.

There is universal acceptance that this condition results in very significant social and psychological handicaps. BDD often starts in adolescence and all the studies that have been carried out have found that people with this condition usually have difficulty in forming and maintaining social relationships. BDD is often associated with social fears and phobias. We also know that many BDD people have more general symptoms of OCD.

A striking feature of people with BDD is that although they may often come across as shy, or very shy, they are, like many anxious people, otherwise in most respects very normal. Many BDD people hold down responsible jobs but at the same time suffer enormous handicaps because of their avoidance of social situations and the psychological distress they experience. The distress associated with the condition leads up to a quarter of people with BDD to attempt suicide.

BDD has been studied by NICE, resulting in guidance being issued (available online at <www.nice.org.uk/cg31>). The guidance recommends psychological treatments (CBT) and medication (high-dose selective serotonin re-uptake inhibitors (SSRIs), such as fluoxetine, in the form of Prozac, for example, are the commonest drugs used). While the results of such treatments are encouraging, in our experience many people are resistant to being treated and very few report a complete, or near complete, recovery, even with the most skilled practitioner. A good treatment outcome for BDD usually means that the distress and handicap caused by the condition is reduced by about 70 per cent. Thus, for most people, it is a lifelong condition. We have met people in their sixties and seventies whose conditions – although slightly improved over the decades – still cause a considerable degree of psychological distress and social restriction.

Morbid jealousy

Morbid jealousy (also known as pathological jealousy) is sometimes seen as one variety of OCD because the person suffers from the repetitive and irrational thought, perhaps that a partner is being unfaithful, and they may therefore engage in a range of compulsive checking behaviours. Morbid jealousy is sometimes called the Othello syndrome; in Shakespeare's play, Othello murders his wife, Desdemona, because of a false belief that she had been unfaithful.

People with morbid jealousy can seek treatment, but it is usually at the request of their partner or due to external agencies becoming involved (such as the police). When one meets a person with morbid jealousy, it is striking that on the one hand they realize that their fears are irrational and that their excessive checking is causing major damage to their relationship. On the other hand they feel compelled to carry on checking and asking their partner for reassurance that they are much loved.

Morbid jealousy may be related to other conditions where obsessive behaviour is demonstrated – for example, stalking. In the classifications of mental health problems, morbid jealousy is included in categories other than OCD. The reason why we mention it in this book is because the treatment methods for morbid jealousy include many of the methods used in the treatment of OCD, notably exposure and response prevention (see Chapter 8).

Sharon

Sharon and her boyfriend Steve had been together for six months. She had a long history of failed relationships, usually as a result of the infidelity of her partner at the time. Over the course of their relationship, Sharon had become increasingly anxious about Steve's 'intentions' and often worried that he may be having an affair. They both attended CBT therapy after Sharon and Steve went to her GP seeking help. On assessment, Sharon explained that whenever Steve was away from the house, she had intrusive thoughts that he 'might be having an affair'. This caused many distressing checking-type behaviours, including telephoning Steve on his mobile approximately 30 times a day (if he didn't answer, Sharon would get herself into an awful state of panic and distress); checking his mobile when he returned home; checking inside his car for any signs of sexual activity (including examining the car carefully for unknown hairs); smelling him for signs of perfume; checking his underwear; cross-examining him about what he did and where he went during the day; refusing to allow him out in the evening (to see friends or to go to the gym); and excessively seeking reassurance that Steve wasn't going to leave her.

Because of her constant need for reassurance from Steve, Sharon had worn him down, and he was finding it difficult to cope with the relationship. He had been thinking lately that it might be best for everyone if he just ended the relationship.

Co-existing mental health problems

As you will now be aware, OCD is an umbrella term that covers a number of related conditions. It can take the form of thoughts (obsessions or ruminations), actions and behaviours (compulsions or rituals), or a mixture of obsessions and compulsions. In all its forms, OCD is commonly associated with a number of other mental health problems, the most common of which (but this is by no means an exclusive list) are depression, social phobia or anxiety, substance abuse, and tics.

Depression

Depression is a common problem in the general population and the figure commonly quoted is that one in five of us will experience a depressive episode during our lives. Therefore, by these chances, one would expect a number of people with OCD to experience depression. Studies have estimated that between 2 and 4 per cent of people in the community have a major depression at any one time. Among people who attend primary care settings, the rate is from 5 to 10 per cent, which rises to 10 to 14 per cent among medical in-patients.

Depression, sometimes called the 'common cold of psychiatry', is the second leading cause of Disability Adjusted Life Years (DALYS), a measure used by the World Health Organization to evaluate the impact an illness has on a person's life. Additionally, WHO has reported that by the year 2020, unipolar major depression will be the leading cause of disability as measured by DALYS. All of us experience a depressed mood at some time. However, when depression lasts for more than a few days, it can disrupt our everyday lives and have a significant impact on our quality of life. It is estimated that such states affect one person in five during their lives.

The term 'depression' covers a wide spectrum of severity. At one end is a condition that, as noted above, is familiar to us all, with feelings of sadness, being 'down in the dumps' and 'can't be bothered' being dominant. At the other end is a condition so severe that the person is in such a state of despair and dejection that he or she 'slows down' in every aspect of life. The person can end up barely able to get out of bed or carry out routine activities of daily living. In such a condition many people have a predominant wish to end their lives.

Depression is no respecter of age, gender, social class, level of intelligence or occupation. In recent years many famous people have 'come out' about depression, and these individuals have done much to defuse the stigma attached to this condition. If you put 'famous people' and 'depression' into an internet search you will find many prominent figures who have had the condition.[3]

However, it appears that depression occurs in people with OCD at a much higher level than could be expected by chance. On the one hand, it seems entirely logical to assume that people whose lives are dominated by obsessions and compulsions will become dejected and feel generally 'down' or depressed because of the impact their problem has on their everyday lives. On the other hand, some people with OCD, even those with the most severe forms, manage to stay very upbeat and positive in their general mood. Others seem to have periods of depression, which appear to be independent of the OCD at that particular time, and these periods of depression may go on for several months but then disappear without any particular reason. To make matters even more complex, some people with OCD only show their OCD when they are in a depressed mood. When their depression lifts, the OCD either reduces in severity or disappears completely.

The relationship between depression and OCD has been studied extensively over the years, and although we know that some people with OCD benefit a great deal from antidepressant medication, both in respect of their OCD and their depression it appears that there is still a great deal to learn about the relationship between these two conditions. However, based on research evidence and our combined experience, if you have a significant level of depression in addition to OCD, you need to seriously consider seeking help for your depression, with either antidepressant medication or psychological treatment, or a combination of the two – in addition to any help you are receiving for OCD. If you notice that depression is a significant problem, you should seek the advice of appropriately qualified professionals; do not try to struggle along alone.

Social phobia or anxiety

Social phobia is sometimes called social anxiety disorder. Social phobia is not just shyness; it is more severe than this. With social phobia people are very anxious about what other people think of them, or how they may be judged by others. As a result, people have great difficulty in social situations, and this can affect their day-to-day life. 'Regular' social anxiety is known to most of us as an uncomfortable feeling of nervousness. Many people have worries about particular social situations, like public speaking or talking to authority figures, or experience more general feelings of shyness or a lack of confidence. For some, however, these social anxieties and fears can become much more troubling and difficult to cope with. Everyday tasks that most people take for granted – such as working, socializing, shopping, speaking on the telephone, and even just going out of the house – might be a wearing ordeal, marked by persistent feelings of anxiety and self-consciousness. Public performances or social gatherings might be out of the question. When social anxiety becomes this severe, people can be diagnosed with social phobia.

Shyness is not a criterion for diagnosis. People differ in how naturally reserved or outgoing they may be, and in regard to the sorts of situations, or people, they might find difficult or be uncomfortable with, individuals who are particularly socially inhibited, avoidant and sensitive to criticism or rejection may meet criteria for avoidant personality disorder. In social phobia, people typically experience excessive feelings of nervousness or dread in relation to feared social situations. They may have specific physical symptoms, such as trembling, rapid breathing, sweating or blushing. At the extreme, panic attacks can occur.

Some people tend to be very self-conscious and worried about whether others might be evaluating them negatively. They often ruminate over past social incidents, worrying about how they might have come across to others. At a deeper level, they can experience chronic insecurity about their relationships with others, hypersensitivity to criticism, or fears of being rejected by others. Many of us go through this kind of experience during adolescence, but for others the problems can persist well beyond those years. Over time, they may come to avoid the situations they fear or become very inhibited or defensive.

Like depression, social anxiety is very common in the general population, but it is found more often than one would expect by chance in people with OCD. Sometimes the social anxiety is connected with the OCD – for example, people may have a concern about behaving (because of their OCD) in a socially inappropriate way, and therefore avoid certain social situations. A person who has a fear of 'blurting out' something inappropriate will find that the simplest way of dealing with this is not to go to parties or any social gatherings if they don't have to. However, social anxiety may be a separate, co-existing problem. Of course, at times the social anxiety and the OCD may interact, making each condition considerably worse. Our advice for anyone with OCD and social anxiety is the same as that for OCD and depression, which is that you may need to seek help for social anxiety as a separate entity, from a suitably qualified health professional.

Substance abuse

People with OCD often seek solace from their anxieties in the use of substances. Twenty or so years ago, the vast majority of people who sought such relief used alcohol. However, with the increasing availability of street drugs in recent years, rising numbers of people use stimulant drugs such as cocaine and amphetamines, or 'downers' such as benzodiazepines, tranquillizers and sleeping tablets. To complicate matters further, it is now not uncommon for people to use a mixture of street drugs and alcohol.

The advice regarding the use of drugs and alcohol with OCD is simple. If your use of substances amounts to anything more than the occasional social drink, then there is a problem. Even with the occasional social drink, your OCD may be made worse. This does not apply to all people with the condition but you need to be aware that alcohol is a depressant drug and it often aggravates OCD symptoms, particularly the next day when the initial pleasant effects have worn off. In our opinion, attempts to control drug and alcohol misuse are futile – the only answer is to aim for total abstinence. We would go so far as to say that, if one continues to use drugs and alcohol in the attempt to deal with the OCD, any treatment will be worthless.

Some people say that if it was not for the OCD, they would not drink or take drugs, and therefore they need treatment for their OCD first. Unfortunately, our knowledge and experiences tell us that this is incorrect. Substance abuse, in all its forms, is a most serious health problem, which can shorten life expectancy, and also destroy families. Therefore, the substance abuse needs to be addressed before the OCD.

Tics

Tics, or abnormal involuntary movements, are sometimes associated with OCD. They can range from minor involuntary movements of particular areas of the body to very noticeable abnormal ones involving many body parts. In its most extreme form it includes compulsions to shout or make noises, a condition known as Tourette's syndrome. Approximately half of the people with Tourette's syndrome have OCD. People with Tourette's syndrome, or those with OCD who have more minor tics, probably suffer from an inborn abnormality in brain structure and there is considerable evidence that this is seen as a genetic condition. Isolated tics are often seen in children with OCD, although these tics may disappear or reduce over time, possibly because the person learns to suppress them.

Anyone with a noticeable tic should always be assessed by a neurologist. Tics are, however, in themselves generally harmless and a neurologist will be able to advise about the use of medications that may assist in their control. In addition, some behavioural treatments have shown good success in the treatment of tics, specifically 'habit reversal' treatment techniques. This treatment relies heavily on helping the person to self-monitor the frequency of the 'habit'; as a sole intervention, it is incredibly successful in its own right.

The overlap between phobias and OCD

Sometimes it can be difficult to distinguish between OCD and a phobia. There is a sense in which most anxious people have an obsession. For example, if you spend all your time worrying about having a panic attack, or finding a spider, then you are obsessed to a certain extent. And you could say that behaviours such as constantly checking a room for spiders have an element of a form of compulsion to them. But there is an extra dimension to OCD, which is the link between the obsessions and the compulsions. A person with OCD usually has a strong feeling that they need to carry out their compulsions or else some dreadful consequence will ensue, and almost always they also feel that they must do their compulsions in a certain way, like a ritual.

A number of phobias appear to be related to OCD and some experts consider certain phobias to be a manifestation of OCD. For example, people with a fear of vomiting (so-called emetophobia) may engage in the obsessive checking of the foodstuffs in their fridge and cupboards, and have a continual obsessive thought about the possibility of vomiting. Such a phobia is quite different from, for example, a fear of spiders, where one might only demonstrate a fear response when one encounters a spider. On the other hand, it is not unknown for people to have a simple phobia, such as spider phobia, to such an extent that they spend most of their waking time thinking about their feared object and engaging in disproportionate amounts of checking behaviour to ensure that they do not come across it. As noted earlier, people can become obsessive about fears of illnesses, such as HIV and

AIDS, and any phobia seen in an excessive form takes on the characteristics of OCD.

In recent years researchers have tried to identify the genetic causes of OCD and phobias, and have suggested that there may be common genetic factors associated with both conditions; hence the overlap that one sees.

4

The causes of OCD and its effects on daily life

The causes of OCD

The causation of OCD is, as we advance in our understanding, becoming increasingly complex. Primarily, the complexity may be due to the probability of there being a number of slightly different disorders under the OCD umbrella, and while some factors may be common to some of these conditions, many cases of OCD may be deemed as having more than one cause. Recent genetic research indicates that OCD may 'run in families', although from generation to generation the form of OCD demonstrated in family members may vary. Some years ago, it was proposed that various mental health problems would be attributable to one single gene, but it now seems likely that a number of genes may be implicated. Some identical twins both have OCD, while in other identical twin pairs, one suffers and one does not. This would lead to the conclusion that genes could not be described as the sole cause.

Examination of the brain and its chemistry is the subject of an enormous amount of research across the world. It seems clear that in some cases the chemical messenger serotonin is involved in the production of symptoms of OCD, and some people seem to benefit greatly from drugs acting on this messenger and the surrounding chemical system. However, others do not benefit from the medication, or may find only partial symptom relief. Recent research using MRI (magnetic resonance imaging) technology shows that some brain structures are overly developed. Sophisticated scanning techniques have demonstrated that the 'hard-wiring' of the brain in some people with OCD differs from the so-called 'normal' population. Various parts of the brain have been implicated, including the orbital cortex and the caudate and cingulated nuclei.

Infection of the brain has also been implicated in the production of

OCD, although research shows that symptoms may disappear within a short time of the infection resolving.

Another issue often highlighted in the findings of research studies is the probability that people can learn their behaviour from others. For example, a child may have a parent with OCD who is continually concerned about the possibility of infection by contaminated foodstuffs, who cleans the fridge and kitchen repetitively and extensively, and continually warns about the dangers of contamination and the need to take precautions against it, such as carrying alcohol gel, and never eating in places that are not of the highest hygienic standards, and so on. It is easy to understand how a child growing up in such an environment may learn obsessional features.

We have thought long and hard about the matter of causation and wish to say two things. First, we believe that it is worth keeping up to date with the results of research, and with the availability of excellent resources on the internet we can learn a great deal about new findings from across the world. Nevertheless, from a practical point of view, becoming preoccupied by what causes one's OCD is not helpful to pursuing a solution. One needs to keep an open mind about causation and, therefore, about treatments, and to remember that most cases of OCD may have several causative influences.

The World Health Organization once ranked OCD as the tenth most disabling illness of any kind in terms of its social and economic impact. OCD-UK, one of the leading charities for OCD, cites on its website (<www.ocduk.org>) the results of economic research, showing that the economic impact of OCD in the USA has been estimated at $8.4m per year. Similar research in the UK indicates a considerable impact here too. Once more, the hidden nature of OCD becomes clear, because although many of those with severe forms of OCD do in fact lose time from work, and this has an impact on national productivity, much of the suffering attributable to OCD is known only to the person themselves and is, therefore, unquantifiable.

Tina
Tina is a 36-year-old librarian who, if she was to describe herself in a few words, would say: 'I have always been a worrier with a great sense of responsibility regarding how my actions might affect others.' Her OCD related to medication – hoarding it and the risk it posed to other people.

Tina went to her GP asking for help for her OCD after the birth of her first child. She explained that while she could deal with the responsibilities of being a mother – and in fact took a leading role in her National Child-birth Trust (NCT) group – she was nevertheless feeling overwhelmed for the first time in her life by her OCD, which she had always managed previously to keep within manageable proportions. On questioning, it appeared that Tina's main problem for many years had been her worry about medications, both over-the-counter and those prescribed for her by her GP.

At first Tina was very guarded in the information she shared, other than to say that she simply could not throw away the packets that contained medication, the product leaflets inside the packets, or indeed any medi-cation that might have been damaged – for example, blister packs. She also said that she was unable to return medication to the pharmacy or the GP surgery for disposal. It soon became clear that Tina's problem with medication was extensive and wide-ranging, and it eventually transpired that she had a number of black rubbish sacks in her loft and garage which were filled by bags within bags within bags(!) containing medication packets, strips of blister packs with no medication in and loose tablets and capsules. None of the medications in these bags were, in relative terms, dangerous – most of the tablets and capsules were par-acetamol, ibuprofen, antibiotics and antihistamines.

Tina also had two large rubbish sacks filled with creams and ointments. Some of these were steroid-based creams she had used for her eczema, but others were simply moisturizers. The problem with these creams was that Tina was worried that she may have somehow 'contaminated' moisturizing creams with the prescribed medication-containing oint-ments. Her major concern was that, somehow, these medications – even in minute quantities – might cause harm to others, and that the empty medication boxes might contain sufficient amounts of medication, such as paracetamol and ibuprofen, to cause liver failure in her nephews and nieces, who quite often visited the house. Later on Tina also mentioned that if she handled the rubbish sacks containing medication, she needed to wear disposable gloves, which after use were put into the garden incinerator. Any contact with medication would also lead to extensive hand-washing.

The treatment that followed Tina's assessment involved demonstrating to her that 'taking risks' with this hoarded medication and the medi-cation packets was reasonable. Following a lengthy period of persuasion, Tina accompanied her therapist to a local shopping centre and, without checking, managed to throw some of the empty medication packets and leaflets into waste bins. Initially this caused her enormous anxiety. However, it demonstrated to her that it was possible to throw away empty medication packets, and 'take the risk' of harming children in the neighbourhood, and this helped Tina to conduct further throwing-away exercises, first in her therapist's company and then as homework on her own. With six sessions of treatment and extensive homework, and employing her husband as a co-therapist, Tina managed to overcome her problem.

Her husband revealed that he would regularly give Tina a great deal of reassurance about throwing things away, but this would be to no avail. On the therapist's advice he began to refrain from giving Tina reassurance and to demonstrate to Tina that he, too, was willing to 'take the risk'. At the end of treatment, Tina volunteered the information that some of the medication packets were more than 20 years old; thus the problem had started during her teenage years. One simple but very pleasing outcome was that Tina and her husband discovered that they had new storage space in their house – an essential with a new baby!

The effects on daily living and quality of life

One question we are often asked is, 'When do you decide that a problem is so severe it needs professional help?' Many people think that this is measured by the severity of the symptoms of that disorder, but a general rule of thumb is to examine the impact that the symptoms have on a person's ability to live a 'normal' day-to-day life of good quality. Thus, the greater the effect on a person's daily functioning or activities of daily living, the more likely it is that they need professional help.

Living with OCD is much like living with other types of chronic illness, like diabetes or asthma; it requires courage, and support from friends, family and co-workers. OCD can have significant effects on the daily life of the person with the condition and those around them. It can be disabling, both mentally and physically. There may be no outward signs, like a raging virus that others can see and understand; and it can eat away at you in the back of your mind nearly every waking moment. Yet most people with OCD suffer in silence, alone, ashamed to tell anyone.

The person who fears that they may have left the gas on in their home, or an electrical appliance on, may have to go back and check numerous times to ensure that everything is off. However, by the time they get back to their car, the thought has reappeared and they again begin to doubt themselves, resulting in further checking. The person who worries about contamination from germs may find it difficult to stop washing in the mornings or when at work. Both of the above will invariably cause the person to be late for work or meetings and appointments.

A person's ability to manage their home (cleaning the house, washing clothes, going to the shops, paying household bills, and so on) may be severely compromised if they have obsessions and compulsions about cleanliness or about locking the front door correctly. Their ability to socialize is likely to be affected. A person's OCD may be such that they find it hard not to ritualize for the period of a few hours when they are out with other people. Knowing this, they may feel embarrassed and ashamed in case others notice it, and decide that perhaps it is better not to go out at all, and stay in instead.

Many CBT therapists use a treatment outcome measure known as the Work and Social Adjustment Scale (WSAS), which was developed and published by Isaac Marks at the Institute of Psychiatry in 1986. The WSAS provides a means of determining the impact that the condition and the symptoms of that condition have upon the client's ability to function in their day-to-day activities. Research has shown that the WSAS has good reliability and validity. It measures five key areas of daily functioning on a scale of 0 to 8, and is rated by both the client and therapist independently of each other (blind to each other). The higher the score, the more the diagnosis/condition has an impact on that specific area of day-to-day functioning.

The five areas measured by the WSAS are (1) home management, (2) work, (3) private leisure, (4) social, and (5) relationships. Usually, your scores are measured at three time periods (this is known as an A-B-A design). Thus, your scores are taken at time period A, which is the baseline period (for example, before treatment starts), at time period B, which is the mid-treatment point, and at time period A again (for example, at the end of treatment – when treatment has finished). What one hopes to see is that while the scores will be moderate to high before any treatment has started (time period A – no treatment), they should be much improved at mid-treatment (time period B – treatment being given), and should have stabilized or stayed the same at the end of treatment (time period C – no treatment).

The evaluation of progress through the measurement of scores, via a questionnaire, is very common in CBT. It is done through the utilization of what is known as a single case experimental design. It is not that dissimilar to the measurement of your temperature, blood pressure, or pulse rate when in hospital or at your local surgery. In a nutshell, the score or measurement (whether your body temperature or your scores on the WSAS) gives you an exact indication of how well you are at a given, specific time period. The idea is that as you improve with treatment (whether that be through antibiotics for an infection or CBT for OCD), you should see your scores or measurements improve with time. If they do not improve, it is crucial that this information is not ignored, and questions should be asked: 'Is my treatment making a difference? If not, why not? What could I do differently?' And so on.

Sometimes it takes a few attempts, trying different strategies, to gain control over the OCD. This in itself is fine, as long as you are able to identify this fact and do something about it (that is, try a different approach). As such it is more important that you try, and if you don't initially succeed, that you are aware of this, than finding the perfect treatment programme first time, every time (which is unlikely). You can download a copy of the WSAS from the internet.[4]

5

Types of intervention and treatment

Evidence-based practice

The philosophical origins of evidence-based practice (EBP) extend back to mid-nineteenth-century Paris and earlier, and it remains a hot topic for clinicians, public health practitioners, purchasers, planners and the public.

EBP is the preferential use of mental and behavioural health interventions or treatments for which systematic, empirical research has provided evidence of statistically significant effectiveness for one treatment over another, as a treatment for specific problems. EBP involves the collection, interpretation and integration of valid, important and applicable patient-reported, clinician-observed and research-derived evidence. The aim of EBP is that the best available evidence, moderated by individual circumstances and preferences, is applied to a person's condition in order to improve the quality of clinical features of evidence-based interventions (EBIs) that must be understood to result in effective use.

EBIs are validated for a specific purpose with a specific population. They are only useful for a certain range of problems and must be paired up with the right person in the right situation. If you randomly match an EBI with a problem it is not designed to address, there is no reason to think that it will work. A hammer is an effective tool, but not with a screw. EBI assumes that the treatment is used in the manner that it was researched. As such, changing parts of an intervention, while not uncommon, can invalidate the EBI. EBIs are typically validated with large group research, or a series of small group studies. While large group research is ideally suited for the documentation of interventions, which typically have a strong effect with a specific problem, it is common that within that large group there are cases where the intervention was not effective. In other words, large group research documents interventions as likely to be effective, not definitely effective, for a specific case. It is critical to remember that even the most effective interventions are often ineffective with some specific cases.

Despite its ancient origins, evidence-based medicine remains a relatively young discipline whose positive impacts are just beginning to be validated,[5] and it will continue to evolve.

Over the past 30 years a great deal of research on OCD has been published. This research has identified the effective and ineffective treatments for OCD. Therefore it is important that the principles of EBP should be applied to the range of interventions used in people with OCD. In this spirit, guidelines have now been published by NICE.

NICE guidelines

The National Institute for Health and Clinical Excellence (NICE) provides guidance, sets quality standards and manages a national database to improve people's health and prevent and treat ill health. NICE makes recommendations to the NHS on new and existing medicines, treatments and procedures, and treating and caring for people with specific diseases and conditions. NICE recommendations are also directed towards local authorities and other organizations in the public, private, voluntary and community sectors on how to improve people's health and prevent illness and disease.

NICE published guidelines entitled *Obsessive-compulsive disorder: core interventions in the treatment of obsessive-compulsive disorder and body dysmorphic disorder* in November 2005 (which can be downloaded from <www.nice.org.uk/cg31>). The guidance was developed to advise on the identification, treatment and management of OCD and BDD.

Although distinct disorders, OCD and BDD share a number of common features and there is a high degree of similarity between the treatments for the two conditions. The guideline recommendations were developed by a multidisciplinary team of healthcare professionals, people with OCD, a carer and guideline methodologists, after consideration of the best available evidence, and are designed for use by clinicians and others providing and planning high-quality care for those with OCD and BDD. There is also an emphasis on the importance of the experience of care for people with OCD and BDD, and carers.

The NICE guideline addresses aspects of service provision, and psychological and pharmacological approaches for those with OCD and BDD from the age of eight upwards. The evidence base is rapidly expanding, and as there are a number of major gaps, future revisions of the guideline will incorporate new scientific evidence as it develops. The full guideline is a staggering 350 pages long and provides in-depth analysis of all the research studies that were carefully examined in making conclusions about which treatments work and don't work. Consequently, it is possible to provide only a brief overview of the NICE guidance within this section. There is also a brief version of the guideline, at 52 pages.

The following are the key recommendations from within the NICE guidance.

For all people with OCD or BDD

Each Primary Care Trust (PCT), mental healthcare trust and children's trust that provides mental health services should have access to a specialist OCD/BDD multidisciplinary team offering age-appropriate care. This team would perform the functions of increasing the skills of mental health professionals in the assessment and evidence-based treatment of people with OCD or BDD, providing high-quality advice, understanding family and developmental needs, and, when appropriate, conducting expert assessment and specialist cognitive behavioural and pharmacological treatment.

OCD and BDD can have a fluctuating or episodic course, or relapse may occur after successful treatment. Therefore, if people who have been successfully treated and discharged are re-referred with further occurrences of OCD or BDD, they should be seen as soon as possible rather than placed on a routine waiting list. For those who have not responded to treatment, care co-ordination (or other suitable processes) should be used at the end of any specific treatment programme to identify any need for continuing support and appropriate services to address it.

For adults with OCD or BDD

In the initial treatment of adults with OCD, low-intensity psychological treatments (including exposure and response prevention – ERP, explained later in the book) – that is, up to ten therapist hours per person – should be offered if the person's degree of functional impairment is mild and/or the person expresses a preference for a low-intensity approach. Low-intensity treatments include:

- brief individual cognitive behavioural therapy (CBT) (including ERP) using structured self-help materials;
- brief individual CBT (including ERP) by telephone;
- group CBT (including ERP).

Adults with OCD with mild functional impairment who are unable to engage in low-intensity CBT (including ERP), or for whom treatment has proved inadequate, should be offered the choice of either a course of a selective serotonin re-uptake inhibitor (SSRI) or more intensive CBT (including ERP) (more than ten therapist hours per person), because these treatments appear to be comparably efficacious. Adults with BDD with moderate functional impairment should be offered the choice of either a course of an SSRI or more intensive individual CBT (including ERP) that addresses key features of BDD.

For children and young people with OCD or BDD

Children and young people with OCD with moderate to severe functional impairment, or those with mild functional impairment for whom guided self-help has been ineffective or refused, should be offered CBT (including ERP) that involves the family or carers and is adapted to suit the developmental age of the child as the treatment of choice. Group or individual formats should be offered depending upon the preference of the child or young person and their family or carers.

Following multidisciplinary review, for children (aged 8–11 years) and young people (aged 12–18 years) with OCD or BDD with moderate to severe functional impairment, if there has not been an adequate response to CBT (including ERP) involving the family or carers, the addition of an SSRI to ongoing psychological treatment 'may be considered' for a child, and 'should be offered' to a young person. Careful monitoring should be undertaken, particularly at the beginning of treatment.

All children and young people with BDD should be offered CBT (including ERP) that involves the family or carers and is adapted to suit the developmental age of the child or young person as first-line treatment.

Stepped care

The clinical effectiveness of psychological therapy (especially CBT) is now widely accepted, but there is a constant dilemma for service providers in attempting to balance the cost of therapy and ensuring an efficient use of limited psychological therapy resources. Current NHS psychological therapy services provide very poor access to effective treatments, with only a minority of people in need able to receive therapy and the vast majority receiving no treatment at all. This is simply because there are not enough trained therapists out there.

A number of authoritative experts have suggested the notion of 'stepped care' as a possible solution and new way of working. Stepped care models have been applied and studied in relation to a range of conditions, including smoking, back pain, alcohol treatment, migraine, anxiety, eating disorders, methadone maintenance, and depression. In stepped care, more intensive treatments are generally reserved for people who do not benefit from simpler, first-line treatments, or for those who can be accurately predicted not to benefit from such treatments. In this way, stepped care has the potential for deriving the greatest benefit from available therapeutic resources.[6]

The NICE OCD and BDD guidance states: 'Stepped care argues that the least intrusive intervention (for example, education or self-help) should be used first, only moving to more intense therapy when less intensive treatment has proved to be insufficiently effective.'

Current interest in stepped care is based on three fundamental assumptions:

- Minimal interventions can provide 'significant health gain', equivalent to that of traditional psychological therapies, at least for a proportion of people (equivalence assumption).
- Using minimal interventions will therefore allow current healthcare resources to be used more efficiently (efficiency assumption).
- Minimal interventions and the stepped care approach are acceptable to people and professionals (acceptability assumption).

The full NICE OCD/BDD guideline concludes:

This guideline suggests that such a model could prove useful if applied to UK settings to encourage access to intensive treatment when severity or risk indicates less intensive treatment would be inappropriate. The Stepped Care Model provides a model for the most effective but least intrusive treatments appropriate to a person's needs. It assumes monitoring of the course of a person's difficulties and referral to the appropriate level of care. Each step introduces additional interventions; the higher steps normally assume interventions in the previous step have been offered for obsessive compulsive disorder and body dysmorphic disorder and/ or attempted, but there are situations where an individual may be referred to any appropriate level. It is suggested that the awareness, recognition and treatment of OCD and BDD proceed across six phases, depending upon need and the characteristics of a person's OCD/BDD. The model also provides a framework to organize services to support the public, people, carers, and healthcare professionals in identifying and accessing the most effective interventions. At all stages of assessment and treatment, families and carers should be involved as appropriate. This is particularly important in the treatment of children and young people with OCD where it may also be helpful to involve others in their network, for example teachers, school health advisers, educational psychologists, and educational social workers.

Medication

Over the years various medications have been used in the treatment of OCD, with varying degrees of success. It seems clear that many medications, such as tranquillizers and beta blockers, are not only not helpful, but distinctly unhelpful. Tranquillizers, for example, have enormous potential for addiction. Similarly, although many people with OCD have disturbed sleep, sleeping medications are not to be recommended, as they do little or nothing to deal with the underlying problem.

There is a great deal of evidence to suggest that a group of antidepressants called selective serotonin re-uptake inhibitors (SSRIs) are very helpful for some people, either alone or in combination with cognitive behavioural therapy. SSRIs work on nerve endings in the brain by increasing the amount of serotonin in nerve cells. As the name implies, the drugs reduce the uptake of serotonin in the nerve cells. Although the mechanism of this action is not exactly understood, it appears that chemical changes effected by these medications change the chemistry of certain pathways in the brain, thus reducing the obsessional anxieties. SSRIs have been subject to a great deal of research across the world and, overall, more than 50 per cent of people with OCD will show significant improvement. In our experience, this improvement ranges from a reduction in anxiety and an increasing ability to cope with obsessions and compulsions, to an almost complete abolition of symptoms in a small minority of people.

It also seems clear that some people who experience only modest improvement with medication may benefit and make more progress if their treatment is combined with cognitive behavioural therapy. In people with the most complex problems, a combination of medication and CBT may be transforming. However, in the same people, either medication or CBT used alone may have little impact.

One difficulty faced by professionals who specialize in the treatment of OCD is predicting who will do well with medication and who will show little or no response. One also needs to take into account the treatment preferences of the individual. Some people will be very reluctant to take medication and will resist any attempts to persuade them to at least give medication a trial. Conversely, others will prefer treatment with medication, rather than embark on a programme of cognitive behavioural therapy. A further difficulty lies in the drugs themselves, as some people do not respond to one variety of SSRI but respond very well to another.

Medication and patient choice

Patient choice is a phrase that can be used too freely and inappropriately. In our experience, people often do not have true, informed choices. In order to make a choice between taking a medication or not, the person needs to know a great deal about what he or she is taking. The treatment of OCD by medication is not something to be taken lightly. If you are going to take medication, you may need to take it for months, if not years, and you therefore need to know something about it. The following are some of the topics that you should find out as much as possible about. This information should be available from the person who prescribes your medication.

- What are the benefits of the medication and what evidence is there for these benefits?
- What are the alternatives, and have the alternatives been compared with the medications you are being prescribed?
- What side effects do these medications have?
- Is this medication associated with any problems following its discontinuation, and if so, what are these problems?
- How often will the medication be reviewed?
- What measures of outcome are to be used? How will the person prescribing know whether you are improving? For example, will a standard questionnaire or rating scale be used?

How long it takes for medications to work

While antidepressant drugs normally start working within a couple of weeks, it takes much longer for the effects of such medications to become evident when used to treat OCD. One issue to bear in mind is that it is often necessary to very slowly increase the dose of SSRIs until an optimum dose (for example, 60mg of fluoxetine) is reached. Once this optimum dose is reached, it can take three months or so for significant benefit to be achieved. At the beginning of treatment with medication, patience is the watchword, and sometimes it is necessary to endure side effects for a few weeks. In the vast majority of cases these side effects diminish and eventually disappear.

How long it is necessary to take medication

As noted elsewhere, the combination of medication with psychological treatment is often the most effective treatment for those with more severe forms of OCD. Once the psychological intervention has been completed, the question that people ask is, 'How long do I need to continue with my medication?' This is a very difficult question, because no long-term studies exist that have followed up people who have successfully completed treatment with a combination of medication and psychological therapy. Therefore one needs to rely on experience, and in our experience, when there is a very long-standing pattern of OCD – rather than an acute episode – coming off medication completely often leads to a relapse. Nevertheless, in most cases medication can be reduced to much lower doses, to reach a 'maintenance dose' that keeps the person well. This process, of finding and reaching a therapeutic dose, which makes an impact on the problem, often takes many weeks.

Follow-up after treatment

As with any problem that requires a great amount of professional input, those who have been successfully treated for a severe form of OCD will probably not want to see their doctors and therapists again, and it is very important for them to return to their normal lives as soon as possible. Nevertheless, it is usual for people to have follow-up sessions, the first perhaps a month after the end of treatment, and then at three-monthly intervals for about a year, and then possibly once or twice a year. This has benefits to both parties.

First, most people feel that it is good to retain contact with professionals who have treated them, 'just in case'. The reality is that a minority will require further treatment in the years ahead. Thus, if people remain in contact with their professional, it should be easier to step back into a treatment process early on, rather than waiting lengthy periods during which time the problem may once more get out of hand. The benefit for the professional of continuing with some form of extended follow-up is the knowledge obtained about the long-term progress, or otherwise, of the individuals who have been treated. In the absence of studies following people for lengthy periods after treatment (an expensive research exercise), such clinical follow-up remains an invaluable way of building our knowledge.

6

Rachel's story

My house is not immaculately tidy and I only wash my hands a few times a day; my clothes are crammed into drawers and the baked beans are never in the same place in my kitchen cupboard. Is this why I lived with the nightmare that is obsessive compulsive disorder for several years before a diagnosis was finally made? Is it because I do not match the stereotypical ideas of how an OCD sufferer behaves? I have OCD, and yet I do not carry out external rituals that draw attention to my disorder: everything takes place in my head, where the 'voice' of this mentally incapacitating illness cannot be heard by others, and where rituals cannot be seen.

OCD manifests itself in many different ways; my symptoms are not uncommon and yet even members of the medical profession failed to recognize them during those early years. They call OCD the 'secret illness', and a lack of diagnosis is common to many people. In my opinion, the reason for this is shared between gaps in understanding and the shame felt by people who are too afraid to reveal the extent of their symptoms. The unwanted thoughts and rituals associated with this disorder are often accompanied by feelings of guilt, whereby those afflicted will blame and punish themselves for its existence. When I look back at my childhood it is apparent that the traits were already there; my father, a very strict clergyman who died when I was 16, encouraged them, although not deliberately. He provided the content with his sermons about the consequences of sin, and everything in our lives had a time and a place; we lived in a world where spontaneity was discouraged and perfection was actively sought. My personal belief is that I was born with an inherent predisposition to OCD, with life experiences providing the catalyst. By the time my first child was born I believed that God would take her away from me because I was so full of sin. This is where the main part of my OCD story begins.

It is impossible to describe the unique love a parent feels for a child.

I felt that love, and yet within weeks of her birth there were times when I could not bear to touch my daughter, and I screamed for her to be taken away. My behaviour was described as rejection, but that description was wrong: it was the behaviour of somebody who felt so undeserving that they were too afraid to embrace their maternal feelings. I do not know which came first, the anxiety that led to the OCD or the clinical depression; I think perhaps they came to me hand in hand. At first I just feared that God would take my daughter away, but then 'magical thinking' – one of OCD's most powerful weapons – came along, and I believed that I had the power to bring about her death with my thoughts. In the early hours of each morning, I would wake abruptly from my drug-induced sleep with the same repetitive, unwanted thoughts in my head. I believed that I could save her if I could make the ruminations go away, but they would not budge – in the same way that a pink elephant will come into your mind if you try not to think about one – and so I tried to replace them by repeating prayers over and over again. Sleep would not return after such a sudden wakening, and so I would wait, panic-stricken, to be told by my mother (who was caring for her at night) that my child had died.

These were my 'groundhog' days and nights when OCD began its vicious circle. It was at a time when psychiatric hospitals would only take mother and baby together, and the local specialist unit was mostly occupied by women suffering from puerperal psychosis. My husband feared for the safety of his new offspring in a world inhabited by people who had completely lost touch with reality, and he did not want us to go. On reflection I believe that I should have been admitted alone, but the word 'bonding' came into every consultation at a time when I most needed rest. My children are now adults and we have an unbreakable bond.

When I look back at my life, many events have been forgotten, and yet I can glance at almost any photograph and recall the subject matter of the current obsession. Without help, OCD people will inadvertently feed their illness and create an environment in which it can thrive. During those early days I would read about sin – even thumbing through the pages of my mother's old edition of the *Encyclopaedia Britannica* – in an attempt to find comforting words; I would also pray obsessively and attend church regularly, even though I believed that my sins would never be forgiven. The concept of hell felt so real that anxiety consumed me and my heart would not stop thumping me from inside. It is hard to describe the fear that severe depression and OCD bring, but imagine waking in the night to find a ghostly figure standing at the end of your bed and then being unable to stop the reactions that are taking place in your body. As always, I tried to replace the thoughts, but if you are as afraid of thinking blasphemous thoughts as I was, one will arrive in your head with the same velocity as the pink elephant.

At that point I could not divulge the contents of my mind to anyone, and the more importance I placed upon the unimportant, the more my OCD gained momentum. I took an overdose two years on from the birth of my daughter, not because I wanted to die – I was too afraid of that – but because I wanted to experience oblivion. I had broken one of the Ten Commandments: nothing juicy, I just believed that I had inadvertently worshipped a false god by trying to learn transcendental meditation in a room in which a picture of a prophet was displayed. It was a significant overdose, which required medical intervention, and although I experienced temporary oblivion, it was not worth it. In our local hospital nurses judged me to the extent that some would not speak to me, the mother of a small child, and the mental torment was so great that I vowed never to repeat the experience.

I did, however, continue to feed my obsession in my attempt to find comfort, and it was at this point that I discovered the concept of an unforgivable sin. It is hard for me to write this, because I am now acutely aware of the distress caused to my family, and I deeply regret my actions, but I was too mentally unwell at the time to make logical decisions. I do not believe that we have the right to judge each other, or that a rational mind can understand the dilemmas of a mind that is overwhelmed by the pain of mental illness.

If you had watched the birth of my second child, almost four years on from a traumatic first experience and the onset of my illness, you would have witnessed a seemingly perfect birth, but all was not as it seemed. As my new daughter was placed in my arms, I tried with all my might to exclude any obsessive thoughts, but they flooded into my mind with great determination and malice; OCD shows no mercy, and particularly loves to destroy the special times. I had been displaying (or should that be hiding?) classic symptoms of OCD, and even though I did not share the specific nature of my fears, I had described those symptoms to professionals on many occasions. I believed that even family members and loved ones would reject me if they could read my mind, and my fear of thinking blasphemous thoughts took over my life as I tried to explain to God that I didn't mean to think them. The type of expletives that some people use in everyday life would taunt my mind, and I felt unclean, but the more I tried to stop them the more they came. It is hard to describe how OCD feels, but I liken it to a chapter in *Alice in Wonderland,* where Alice is in the White Rabbit's house and has grown so big that she fills the room; the thoughts grow and grow until they seem to occupy an entire mind, pressing against the inside of your head until it hurts and the depression is all-consuming.

Not all my obsessions have been of a religious nature, although these are the ones I fear the most. The sound of a dog barking can fill my head, even when it is silent, and I once became so preoccupied by an unaligned steering wheel that I could think of nothing else for the duration of a holiday; the much used scratched record analogy is very befitting. Some obsessions are part of me (for example, I have mentally calculated my daily calorie intake several times a day since I was a teenager) and they do not cause distress, so I leave them alone. I do not believe that we should or can confront everything, only those obsessions that have an unacceptably negative impact on our lives or lead us to avoid situations. Avoiding staying in hotel rooms for a large part of my life because of my fear of the Bible only intensified that fear and led to further avoidance and anxiety; this could only be reduced by exposure therapy.

There have been many times in my life when others have mistaken my rational thoughts for irrational ones; as hard as it is to comprehend, people with OCD tend to know when they are being irrational and have a good understanding of what is real. This is something I will never be able to comprehend fully or explain, but it was highlighted when a stalker came into my life and did not leave for five years. He was a neighbour with learning difficulties, and while I understood that he was not a threat, I could not bear being constantly followed and watched. My reactions were extreme, and obsessive thoughts and behaviours took over, but on this occasion my history of OCD meant that others found it hard to differentiate between obsessive and 'normal' fears.

Within a year I had been hospitalized and was receiving drug treatment and electroconvulsive therapy. Shortly after I had been discharged I suffered a drug-induced seizure in the middle of the night. Having been unconscious for 20 minutes, I woke up feeling confused and frightened, and yet I still looked at the neighbour's window in my ritualistic way, and thought of nothing else but him as I was taken into the ambulance. Such is the power of obsessive thoughts that not even this, or the birth of my child or being at my mother's deathbed, could stop them.

The story I have told you so far provides a lesson in how not to deal with OCD. Four years after this incapacitating disorder took over my life, I was fortunate to see a psychologist with a special interest in OCD; he guided me in the right direction. He was horrified when I first told him my thoughts, and ejected me from the room saying that I was evil and beyond help; I could see in his eyes that I disgusted him. Of course, that is not what *really* happened – that is what my obsessive mind told me *would* happen. In reality I saw the corners of his mouth move towards a smile as I voiced my unwanted thoughts (expletives and all), and his eyes told me that he had heard it all a thousand times before. The psychologist had begun the long task of desensitizing my thoughts through exposure therapy.

The first time I said my most feared phrase, he let me put it into context by saying, 'This is an unwanted thought' (in case God did not realize). This is called 'safety behaviour' – the equivalent of crossing your fingers behind your back – and I was to use it and get away with it many years later in a group session with a far less experienced therapist. The second time, he told me to put my words in context after saying them, but then he stopped me from doing so. Fear shot through me at that moment, but OCD cannot be conquered without putting yourself in the situations you fear most, and I have been in all of them. If fear is in your path you must walk through it, not round it, to achieve your goals. For me it was not just a case of saying the thoughts out loud once, I had to repeat them over and over again, and even record them so that I could play them back to myself.

My illness did not go away – I will always have an obsessive mind, and that can also bring gifts – but cognitive behavioural therapy unlocked some of the doors where the thoughts and fears had been trapped, and my life began to change. Sadly, two years after my first course of CBT I was back at the hospital and it was at this time that electroconvulsive therapy was seen as the best course of treatment for my anxiety and depression. SSRI medications were yet to be made available, but now, more than two decades later, I am fully aware of their importance. I went without medication for 15 years following the seizure, and lived with a deep-seated fear of taking antidepressants, but now they work alongside CBT and I lead a far more fulfilling life, where I can express my creativity.

It was a further bout of severe depression and OCD in 2007 that took me back along the road to a specialist unit in north London, but this time I emerged with more understanding and sufficient strength to make significant changes to my life; I finally took responsibility for my own life and learned to stop the constant requests for reassurance on which OCD feeds. I could not have done this without the help of my psychologist, who has played a leading role in the story of my life since I first met him in 1989, or without the aid of the SSRI fluoxetine. I am not cured, because you cannot cure a personality, but I now face my fears, share my experiences and use my obsessive mind to feed my creativity. It was the concept of 'action before motivation' that helped me on my way. There are many theories as to the causes of OCD, some of which have been backed up by the results of brain scans, but I feel certain that a hormonal imbalance has played a major part in my story.

Depression and OCD destroy motivation and often lead to inactivity and a constant need to seek reassurance. It is important to break the cycle, and this is why the concept of 'action before motivation' remains an important part of my life, and why I have had to learn not to feed my OCD with endless requests for reassurance. It is the abnormal demands to which I am referring: questions like, 'I'm not a bad person, am I?' or, 'I won't go to hell, will I?' If a person's OCD takes the form of body dysmorphia there is no point in telling that person that they are attractive, because they will not believe you, or the other hundred people who have told them. On the contrary, OCD thrives on the reassurances of others, because they discourage the sufferer from seeking the strength we all have within us. As with safety behaviours, I became an expert in tricking people into providing me with reassurances; even after those around me had been instructed not to respond to my persistent requests, I was devious and managed to extract them.

Action, in my case, involved regular exercise and the pursuit of my creative hobbies when my mind was trying to persuade my body to lie on the bed and wallow; the former is difficult when energy has been depleted through a lack of sleep, but I persisted. At the hospital, each day would begin with a behavioural activation session, during which we would all agree on our targets for the day. As always, my camera played a major part in this, and I would often make a pledge to take photographs in the park during the lunchtimes, even though the desire was missing. It was on one such occasion that I met my friend, the kestrel, which seemed unafraid of me and posed beautifully on a tree that was covered in dark red leaves. He seemed to absorb my OCD for a few short minutes, but in time and with a great deal of perseverance, minutes can turn to hours.

I have met many OCD people during my long association with the hospital and I have liked them all. The vast majority have been gentle, caring and compassionate, with an overdeveloped conscience and a desire to make the world a better place. I would not put myself in that category, but others do. Like me, many of them have been the victims of faulty thinking, such as mind-reading, catastrophizing and magical thinking; my mind-reading still leads me to imagine that others are thinking negative thoughts about me, but I have learned to accept this.

Sitting in a room full of people who are describing their obsessions and carrying out exposure therapy is a surreal experience; in your heart you know that nothing you or anyone else is saying makes sense, but all you can hear are the words of your OCD. Some people cannot bring themselves to touch anyone or anything, and sit with fists clenched in front of their chests. They cannot open doors with their hands or touch their body or clothing, for fear of contamination. Believing that they will be responsible for the death of loved ones, I have heard hospitalized young women plead for visits from home to be cancelled. Many feel so unclean that no amount of washing can ever cleanse them. To be told to touch something, or not to wash their hands (with taps in some cases turned on by elbows), can cause terrifying anxiety. But like all of us whose lives have been blighted by this disorder, they can only work towards recovery if they face their fears head on, and learn not to be afraid of fear itself.

The rituals associated with OCD are usually quite bizarre, but most people feel certain that bad things will happen if they fail to carry them out. To watch somebody being told not to act out a compulsion is by no means easy; it is difficult to witness the reactions of a young person who truly believes that his family have just been killed in a car crash, because he has not followed an uninvited thought with an action, such as banging a table with his knees. I have met some for whom external rituals occupy up to 20 hours a day, with lives dominated by compulsions such as counting, reciting, checking, perfecting, ordering, cleaning, touching, or not touching, as the case may be. Each person's illness bears its own trademark, although there are usually common themes. Some people, like me, can function in the real world (most of the time) because the obsessions and rituals take place in their heads, but others cannot.

Exposure therapy is a vital component in the battle against OCD, but it does not bring the same immediate relief and satisfaction as exposure to the object of a phobia, because an obsessive compulsive fear is far more complex. When I, a serious arachnophobe, held a spider at the end of an exposure session at London Zoo, I experienced a degree of elation, because fear was the only item on the agenda and I had been able to eliminate a large amount of it. The battle against OCD is far slower, but it can be won and life can be rich and fulfilling. As for reasoning with an OCD mind, that does not come into the equation because rationality cannot begin to compete against irrationality. I feel as if these two areas of my mind are too far away from each other to interact, and yet, as I have expressed before, I can still hear the rational part. Is it any wonder that the World Health Organization lists OCD as one of the top ten most debilitating illnesses?

An overpowering fear of being judged and labelled has led to secrecy in my life. When I started writing a blog on my personal website (<www.rachelpiper.me.uk>), I was eager not to give anything away, but I slowly realized that I was doing nothing to help rid the world of stigmas by hiding my own illness. Writing openly about clinical depression and OCD has been a major exposure for me, but as with all exposures it has helped me move forward and I have become stronger. It has also helped others, for which I am thankful. I am so much more than my illness and I feel comforted by the fact that my website tells the bigger picture, with an insight into my creative mind and the way in which I use humour as a tool to get me through some of life's difficult moments.

Humour in the treatment of mental illness can cause controversy: another OCD sufferer and I once got 'told off' at the hospital for laughing at our own afflictions. The therapist informed us that OCD 'is not a laughing matter', but I, and the more experienced professionals, do not agree. The psychologist who has treated me over the years will joke about some of the subjects of my obsessions, but he is laughing with me and he knows when he can use humour and with whom. I believe that the 'O' in OCD can be channelled creatively, and I do not believe that I would have achieved as much without this element of my personality. It is only in recent years that I have started sharing my creative output with the world; I would often feel too insecure to do so in the past and it could take me hours to prepare and mount a single piece of work. The perfectionist in me can be a ruthless quality controller.

Following my latest period of treatment, I set myself tasks that took me out of my comfort zone. I wanted to help change the world, so I looked at the skills I have got, rather than the ones I wished I had. One of my greatest challenges was prompted by the words in an email, which described life at the bottom of the economic pyramid and the work of the charity WaterAid. My initial feelings were of inadequacy, because like many people I wished that there was something I could do, and it felt as if the proverbial light bulb had illuminated above my head when I realized that there was. Sometimes we look too far away from ourselves when we think about what we have to offer, but at this point my creative mind took over and I decided that I would sell my photographs for the charity.

Putting yourself in the spotlight when you do not feel confident is not easy, but as with OCD fears, the more you do it the wider your comfort zone becomes. My desire to help others who suffer from OCD and depression has also been satisfied in this way; up until this point my thinking had been very narrow, but I realized that there were ways of helping other than offering direct counselling, and so I decided to have a sale at the hospital where I received treatment, and at the 2008 OCD Action Conference, to raise money for the latter. I work with charities because I want to, not because I am trying to prove to God or myself that I am a good person; this is very important.

I often photograph spiders these days, and I get as close as I can with my macro lens; when I see the results I am reminded that fear can be overcome. I draw with coloured pencils now, and I no longer say to myself, 'I can't draw', because I can. If somebody admires my work I just say, 'Thank you'; I had to teach myself to do that, rather than point to a fault that nobody else had noticed. Our minds listen to the words we say and negative words can feed low self-esteem. Creativity provides an outlet for my obsessive mind, and my perfectionist tendencies (annoying as they sometimes are) also play their part.

In my opinion, our journeys should not be about overcoming OCD, but about working towards finding acceptable levels and using every-thing we have inside us. I often encounter people who say that they haven't got time or they don't feel mentally prepared to embark upon something new, but I feel that 'now' is the best time to start; we can always find time, even if it means getting up an hour earlier or missing a soap opera on the television. Displaying my creative work was very difficult at first; I would spend hours preparing each piece and the fear of being judged incompetent or arrogant would often be a great hin-drance. Those fears remain to a lesser extent, but I continue to show my art to the world and I have been successful in international photo-graphic competitions and in raising money for various charities.

Before I finish my story, I would like to introduce you to Oscar Charlie Delta. Oscar is the name I have given to the character that personifies my OCD; in illustrating Oscar I depicted him as a dark thought bubble with a mouth and eyes, but in reality he is just the sound of the negative inner voice over which I have no control. I have published the story of Oscar on my website (<www.rachelpiper.me.uk/oscar.html>), in which he is not just the character that infiltrates my mind, but the persecutor of every OCD sufferer. He represents the constant intrusive thoughts, urges and images that cannot be ignored, and the compulsions and rituals that those with OCD are driven to repeat to keep themselves and those around them safe.

I believe that all people who suffer from OCD have the strength within them to move forward and lead a fulfilling life. I live my life a day at a time and I believe that I am who I am at each point in my life. There is no point in mourning who I could have been or regretting the events of the past; confronting my fears has provided me with the strength to be who I am today, and my obsessive nature brings with it the gift of creativity. I still practise 'action before motivation' when I am feeling low, and if Oscar tries to torment me with his cruel words I write about the experience, rather than conceal it. There is nothing that cannot be shared, although it is important to share your thoughts with the right person: somebody who understands that the thoughts are only there because they are so abhorrent to you. Sitting among fellow OCD people, I know that the man who is tormented by images of himself abusing his child could never do so, or that the woman who constantly imagines pushing a fellow passenger in front of a train is incapable of deliberate harm, but not everybody understands OCD.

A great deal has been written about SSRIs, particularly on the internet, and in my opinion much of the information presented is neither factual nor helpful. I am glad that I listened to professional advice, as my perseverance during the initial period of bodily adjustment has led to greater fulfilment. SSRIs are an important part of my life, and they are likely to remain so, but for me they are not the solution; I combine them with regular exercise, exposure therapy when required, the philosophy of action before motivation and the pursuit of many creative activities. When fear stands in my way I try to walk through it, because if I remain stationary or walk round it I know that I am handing power to Oscar.

OCD is a misunderstood and incapacitating illness, but I am encouraged by the changes that I have witnessed since my story began. The emergence of new understanding and research, more effective medications and the development of more OCD-specific cognitive behaviour therapies have all helped in a battle which we will continue to fight. For many years I tried to find all the answers, but now I accept that sometimes there are none. I concentrate on what I know I believe, not what I think I should, and my fundamental beliefs are that we should look after our world and respect our fellow human beings and the creatures that inhabit it. A strict religious upbringing introduced me to the concept of sin at a very early age and the emergence of severe OCD heightened my inherited quest to seek perfection; I was looking for certainty, but to live with this illness we need to accept uncertainty. I admire and respect people who have faith, but I believe that children should feel safe and should not be exposed to fearful religious concepts.

To all those who suffer from OCD, please take comfort in the fact that you are not alone. Recovery is about teamwork. We need others in our quest, but ultimately we must draw strength from within and face our fears; we all have that strength.

Part 2
Treatment and self-help

7

Defining your problem and selecting goals

Although it may seem rather obvious, defining the precise nature of your problem is the first necessary step on the road to recovery. Taking the example of someone overwhelmed with financial problems, you might imagine that they reach a point when they no longer open letters from creditors, and leave them in a pile in a drawer. Eventually, one of the creditors will ask for the owed money, thus causing even more worry about the problem. In this situation the person can only get to grips with their difficulties by, first of all, establishing how much money is owed, and to which creditor. Once this is identified, the next step is to calculate the income and assets from which debts might be paid. It might then be established which debts should be seen as priorities over others – for example, the mortgage might be considered the most essential payment to meet, while other debts, such as a loan from a friend who has already said that they can wait, might be put to one side to be paid later.

Although this analogy does not exactly match the problems encountered by a person with OCD, the essential principles are the same. You need to work out the components of your problem, in order to establish the severity of the components (that is, the obsessions or compulsions), then decide what needs to be tackled first. You could also make a list of factors that might make the problem better or worse, so that it can be seen exactly how problems are maintained. In carrying out this exercise, you might observe that seeking reassurance works in the short term but not in the long term, and that avoiding a particular situation provides immediate relief but in the long term intensifies fears. You might also see that drugs or alcohol can reduce anxiety but at the same time identify an increasing reliance on these substances.

It might be helpful to attempt to break down the problem in this way:

- Use the categories set out in Chapter 2 to identify obsessions, compulsions, or a mixture of obsessions and compulsions.
- Organize the obsessions and compulsions in themes – for example, obsessive thoughts, repetitive actions, need for symmetry.
- Make a list of how problems affect your daily life and activities and the reason why. For example, 'I avoid going to the cinema in case I hear or see something that triggers my sexual obsessions', or, 'I avoid travelling by public transport because of the fear of coming into contact with what I think might be dried blood.'
- Try to rate each of the problems listed on a scale of 0 to 100, when 0 is no problem and 100 is the worst possible problem; or alternatively, 0 means that the problem gives no distress/upset and 100 means that the problem gives the most intense distress/upset imaginable. One word of warning here: be comprehensive in respect of providing yourself with a picture on paper of all aspects of your problem, but on the other hand, your problem lists do not need to be in so much detail that you have written a book! People with OCD often have the need to be very precise in everything that they do and this may extend to the definition of your problems. The advice here is to undertake this exercise realizing that you might miss out certain details. The important, central objective is to obtain a general picture. Taking the example of a car, one might want to draw body, wheels, doors and headlights, but would not necessarily need to have a working diagram of each and every circuit board or working part!

Selecting targets or goals

As with the psychological treatment, the question you first need to ask yourself is, 'What would I like to do that I can't do at present because of my problems?' Try to answer this question honestly. Be selfish; think about what you want, putting to one side what you think others might expect of you. For example, you might want to leave home for work in the morning without spending half an hour checking doors, windows and locks. Therefore, your goal would be to leave home, making sure by checking once that all the doors and windows are closed and the burglar alarm is on. On the other hand, you might think that you should endeavour to be less concerned with order and symmetry and you might say, 'Although I realize that order and symmetry may be a problem for others, it is definitely not a problem for me. I don't spend huge amounts of time making my house just so!' If this is the case, order and symmetry should not be selected as your targets, as these issues are not a problem for you.

Compulsions that take the form of observable behaviours, such as cleaning, washing, checking and repeating, obviously lend themselves very easily to target-setting; targets can be selected about the time one takes to carry out a certain action, the number of times one performs an activity, and so on. Setting targets for obsessions, however, is sometimes more of a problem, although there are ways of doing this.

For example, someone who has particularly aggressive obsessions and who avoids situations where these obsessions might be triggered, might select confronting that situation and experiencing the obsession. Someone with a religious obsession, whose thoughts are similar to those of Madeline in Chapter 1 (who could not help combining a sexual thought or image with the name of Christ), could select as a target being able to stand outside a cinema showing a particularly sexual film and to tolerate the discomfort involved. The target might also include being able to say to yourself at the same time, 'Standing here brings to mind various sexual thoughts and images. This is all part of my OCD. It has no consequence to the life that I lead and I try to lead a life based on a particular moral and ethical code. So standing here in this situation is, in itself, harmless. I will face my feared thoughts for as long as it takes for those thoughts to disappear.' Or someone might aim to tolerate the discomfort they feel when hearing unusual noises, words or music, for as long as it takes for the distress involved to subside.

All targets should be selected with an overall goal of working towards a pattern of life activities that you consider to be 'normal' (everyone's definition of normal is different!). As noted above, target behaviours should be linked to what you want, not what others want. Therefore, in the case of problems associated with noise, selecting a target of tolerating the sounds of a football crowd will not help in your endeavour to conquer your obsession with noise if you are not a football fan. You might have more success if one of your interests is politics and you select to attend noisy political meetings as a target.

It will help if you ensure that the goals you select are *functional objectives* rather than being based upon *symptom reduction*. Goals should be SMART, an acronym that stands for:

- Specific
- Measurable
- Achievable
- Realistic
- Time-based.

Goals should detail what you will be able to achieve if the symptoms have been addressed. Try to ensure that all goals meet the SMART criteria. Examples might be as follows.

Short-term goals (within one to two months of treatment)
- To increase daily activities within the home, including basic household duties such as washing and ironing, resuming a daily routine of activities for up to one hour in total a day, and to aim to complete two hours of these activities per day.
- To increase daily activities outside of the home, including going for a 20-minute walk on a daily basis.
- To increase your level of social interaction, to include meeting with friends for lunch at least once a week.

Long-term goals (within three to six months of treatment)
- To resume travel as a driver or passenger on longer outings, including trips to the coast or countryside once a month.
- To resume gym attendance on a once-a-week basis.
- To resume full, normal social activities. including regular (at least weekly) lunch and evening meetings with friends and family.
- To meet with your employers within a certain number of weeks in order to explore return to work options and possibilities.

Developing your treatment plan

Your plan should involve using those methods which years of research have shown to be the most important for overcoming OCD. There are two central approaches that have been shown to be effective. Combined, these two approaches form the basis of cognitive behavioural therapy. They are exposure and response prevention, and cognitive strategies, to which we turn in the next chapters. Although cognitive behavioural therapy may also include other methods, such as having the family help you, these two approaches form the focus of any reasonable treatment programme; these approaches may, or may not, be facilitated by the use of medications (described in Chapter 5).

8

Exposure and response prevention

Exposure

We set out in the following pages a number of strategies that may be used to overcome OCD, and central to these strategies is the principle of exposure. Obsessions and compulsions are fundamentally grounded in a fear – for example, a fear that if you do not wash your hands, you will catch a deadly disease or transmit contamination to others; a fear that you will commit an act of gross indecency if you are close to a child; a fear that you will be responsible for harm coming to others. Over the past 50 years or so it has become clear that in order to reduce a fear, one needs exposure to that fear.

Thus, in the simple example of a phobia of spiders, you need to face spiders – perhaps starting with photographs, then spiders in a sealed jar, until you are comfortable with a spider crawling on your hand. Such a phobia will not respond very well if you are immediately asked to put a tarantula in the palm of your hand (this is known as 'flooding'); exposure needs to be graded – people need to face difficult, but just about manageable, exposure tasks, one at a time, to overcome their fear. Similarly, if you have a fear of public places, you would not start treatment with a trip to a busy shopping centre at Christmas; rather, you might begin by being accompanied on a walk down your own road at a quiet time of day.

This approach to fears and phobias has been very thoroughly researched and there are literally thousands of accounts of successful research studies in support of exposure.

What we know about exposure and the best way to employ it

First, as noted above, exposure needs to be gradual and you need to feel that you are able to undertake the task that you have set for yourself, whether you are doing so with the help of a therapist, with the help of a friend or family member, or on your own. We know that exposure needs to be prolonged. Simply put, you need time to gradually allow yourself to get used to the anxiety/fear that the exposure will inevitably cause, in allowing the body's responses to fear to reduce gradually. This may take anything from a few minutes up to several hours, although usually one hour is sufficient. What is very important is that once you start your exposure task, you don't 'escape' it before your anxiety starts to naturally reduce; to do this will result in what is known as 'sensitization', or an increase in fear/anxiety. For this reason, you need to pick an exposure task that you know you will be able to 'stay with' without needing to escape.

The main 'learning theory' that underpins the fear reduction seen during exposure is that of 'habituation'. Habituation is the term used when a person's response to a stimulus gradually diminishes with repeated exposure to that stimulus.[7] There is little disagreement across dictionaries about habituation definitions; the *Concise Oxford Dictionary* defines habituation as 'to make or become used to something'; *Encarta* defines it as 'to make somebody used to something: to accustom a person or animal to something through prolonged and regular exposure', while *Merriam-Webster* has 'a decrease in responsiveness upon repeated exposure to a stimulus'.

This form of learning is usually outside of 'consciousness' and naturally occurs. Every day, non-anxious habituation episodes might include the process of 'getting used' to living next to a noisy road, railway line or flight path (over time, one gets used to the noise); or getting used to certain smells in work or the family home (for example, smells associated with cooking, which one might notice on entering the house, but not be aware of after 10 or 20 minutes). Habituation to the physiological effects of drugs is one key theory of explaining why a drug user requires increasing amounts of the same drug, over time, in order to gain the same physiological result.

Habituation is considered important in the area of sensory processing, as it allows 'filtering' of less important (less novel) information received from the surrounding environment, which means that one can focus on the novel elements. Figure 8.1, overleaf, shows the usual habituation that is observed when using exposure; the uppermost line shows the first exposure, the lowest line the final exposure trial. With repeated exposure to an anxiety-provoking stimulus (such as driving on a motorway in the rain), the anxiety response slowly wanes over time.

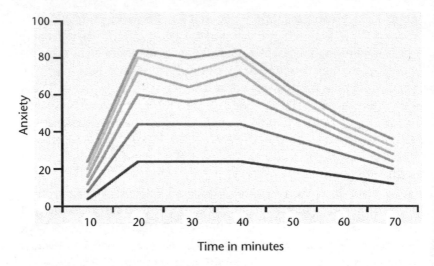

Figure 8.1 An exposure graph

An effective exposure programme

A number of factors are likely to improve the effectiveness of an exposure programme.

Making a plan before embarking on an exposure programme is important, bearing in mind that exposure may take many days, weeks or even months to achieve its eventual goal. Under this plan exposure sessions should be conducted frequently – once a week is not likely to be effective, and daily exposure is the best.

As to the length of exposure, you need to expose yourself to that which causes distress for as long as it takes for that fear to begin to diminish. As time goes on, you will see that anxiety reduces over time, from session to session. The rule of thumb is to say that the longer the session of exposure the better, and research shows that a session lasting two hours turns out to be much better than four sessions of 30 minutes.

Exposure can be carried out in the imagination as well as in real life, and sometimes this is a good way of preparing yourself. Thus, for example, in the case of John (see page 75) touching the waste paper bin, he might simply sit and visualize carrying out this task. Imaginal exposure can be carried out as a preliminary activity, and may be very helpful in assisting you to prepare for something that, at present, you cannot contemplate undertaking in real life.

Gradation is also important. As we have said, conducting exposure in graded doses of difficulty is the best way of proceeding. Trying to tackle the unmanageable may lead to failure and feelings of dejection. When making your plan, you might be able to decide on the steps you can contemplate taking. Plans need to be revised at intervals and it might be worthwhile looking at your plan and progress on a weekly basis.

Having a co-therapist, perhaps a family member or friend, who understands the problem and has an idea of the principles of treatment (perhaps ask them to read this book first) will be helpful for most people. This book may also be useful if you are undergoing therapy from a professional. You could use it, and perhaps others that follow a cognitive behavioural approach, to help guide you between your treatment sessions.

One question that we are often asked is, 'Is it necessary to experience anxiety during exposure sessions?' When confronting situations after many years of avoidance, some people find that their exposure is much easier than they imagined and they experience little, or no, distress. This is definitely not a problem. Sometimes, anticipation of therapy is much worse than the therapy itself.

Anxiety, avoidance and escape

While it may never be ascertained as to exactly why a person develops an anxiety disorder, it is possible to see what 'maintains' anxiety or keeps it going. Invariably, there are two main reasons. The first is avoidance and the second is escape. A person with a fear of something will tend to gradually develop avoidances (so they do not have to face their anxiety), or should that fail, escape (allowing them to remove themselves from the situation).

Avoidance is often obvious and is a good indicator of the nature of the anxiety disorder, as different disorders have slightly varying avoidance profiles. It is worth noting that people can avoid in two ways: in real life and in the imagination. While you may be behaviourally exposing yourself to a fear, you may be cognitively avoiding. For example, if you have a social phobia (a fear of being negatively appraised by others) you might put yourself in a social situation, but you are cognitively trying to distract yourself from that situation (perhaps imagining that you are on a nice secluded beach, or counting to 100 in your head).

It is also possible to avoid within an exposure. So while you may be in a social situation (in a bar at lunchtime), you may still be avoiding, by wearing sunglasses (to avoid eye contact), listening to music through earphones (to avoid conversation, hearing your environment), or reading a newspaper (avoiding the possibility of social contact). When going to the bar, you may have the exact money, so as to avoid having to wait for change and increase the likelihood of conversation. You may make sure that you are sitting as close to an exit as possible so that you can 'escape'; it may also be the least busy exit. If you are fearful of public transport, you may be more likely to sit downstairs on a bus, as close as possible to the doors, or even to stand near the doors, than take a seat upstairs or at the back of the bus.

When thinking about your OCD, it is important to understand your avoidances and escape behaviours. Sometimes these are obvious, but sometimes they can be very subtle. Use an anxiety diary for a couple of weeks, as this can often give a good indication of current avoidance and escape behaviours. The diary should include information about the anxieties encountered, describing what caused the anxiety, what thoughts you had, and what responses you made (for example, hand-washing). It is also helpful to quantify how severe the anxiety was, using a scale of 0 to 10 (0 = no anxiety, 10 = worst imaginable).

How exposure therapy is delivered

Exposure therapy can be delivered in two separate ways: *in vivo* (live), and imaginal (in the imagination).

In vivo exposure

In vivo or live exposure involves you being assisted to face your avoided fears in real life. A structured way of doing this is the use of a fear hierarchy, in which you list all your avoidances, then rate each item in order of difficulty, from 0 for 'not difficult' to 100 for 'unable to do this'. A series of homework targets can be compiled for you to work on, on a daily basis, beginning with the easiest things; as you get used to each one, you can gradually move up to the next item on the hierarchy.

Imaginal exposure

Imaginal exposure involves facing your avoided fears in your imagination. This is very important with OCD, as the obsessional thought, image or impulse will be in the imagination and not outwardly observable. You list all your distressing thoughts, images and urges, again creating a hierarchy, and then expose yourself gradually to them, in your own imagination. You do this simply by repeatedly thinking about the distressing thought, image or impulse, until you get used to it (become habituated to it).

The principles of exposure

The four main principles underlying effective exposure are that it needs to be graded, focused, prolonged and repeated.

- *Graded* – you are encouraged to face your fears in a graded way, starting with something that you believe you can achieve, and gradually increasing the level of exposure as you have success at given targets.
- *Focused* – you are focusing upon or cognitively engaging with the feared situation to which you are exposing yourself. To enhance this you might be asked to describe your surroundings and what you are doing to yourself in your mind during your exposure.
- *Prolonged* – the exposure should last long enough for you to begin to at least get used to your anxiety. It could be anything from a few minutes to more than an hour; it is important that the exposure is long enough for your anxiety to begin to decrease. If you are undertaking exposure with the help of a therapist, a session will usually be set at one hour. Some fears don't lend themselves to the possibility of being continually exposed to them for a certain length of time. For example, if you fear meeting new people for the first time, you might be asked to experience several frequent exposures over the space of an hour, perhaps by going out into your shopping centre every lunchtime and approaching different strangers and asking them the time. Your aim might be to approach ten people during that hour.
- *Repeated* – the exposure should be repeated regularly, which usually means daily. A good combination of the principles of prolonged exposure with repeated exposure, might be that exposure is done for an hour every day.

Response prevention

Exposure and response prevention (ERP) is a treatment that was developed more than 40 years ago; it was the first effective psychological treatment for OCD.

Consider the rituals that you employ when you have an obsessive thought – these are attempts to 'escape' the anxiety that your thought causes you. For example, if you have a thought that you are contaminated, and may pass on your 'germs' to others, then you will become highly anxious. By ritualizing (such as thorough hand-washing), you are trying to cancel out the thought and the anxiety – thus 'escaping' the anxiety.

This escape behaviour stops you 'habituating' to the stimulus or trigger, because you do not give yourself the chance to 'naturally' get used to the anxiety, thus letting it go away by itself. Furthermore, the ritual gives you 'short-term' relief from the anxiety-provoking thought, as it cancels it out. While this may be helpful at the time, you become more and more reliant on this, thereby learning that only through ritualizing can you stop your anxiety, and so becoming intolerant of other ways of trying to address the anxiety. In learning theory literature, this is called negative reinforcement.

Doing the ritual might result in short-term relief from the anxiety, at that precise moment, but it doesn't get rid of the problem. Next time you have a similar thought, you rely upon your ritual to help you through that immediate anxiety. This can be viewed as a form of 'coping', and while it helps you to cope for that period in time, it does not treat the underlying problem: the anxiety that the thought causes.

Response prevention is basically a strategy to help people overcome their natural habit of wanting to ritualize. The effect of the ritual is that it probably reduces the anxiety at that time, and thus achieves its objective. Response prevention attempts to try to stop the ritual giving relief, reduce the negative reinforcement that is occurring, and break the dependence or habit of using only one means of behaving as a way of coping. The aim is for someone's anxiety to reduce naturally – not unnaturally, through using a ritual, as the ritual stops the natural recovery involved in habituation. Therefore, response prevention attempts to cancel out the effect of the ritual, straight away, by the development of methods to reintroduce the original thought and the anxiety this causes.

For example, if you have a thought that your hands are contaminated and that you may pass germs on to others, then you will be inclined to wash your hands. Response prevention would attempt to cancel this out by asking you to 're-contaminate' your hands immediately (perhaps by touching the carpet near the door, or touching the toilet door handle). Thus the effect that the washing provided is cancelled out.

Or you might have a thought that you might stab your family if the knives are not locked away. You then lock the knives away and repeat to yourself, 'It's ok – I'm safe, the knives are locked away.' Response prevention would involve asking you to unlock drawer with the knives in, and repeatedly say to yourself, 'The knives are not locked away and I feel unsafe.'

Thus response prevention attempts to encourage you to 'stay with' your anxiety so that you can naturally get used to it (habituation), by cancelling out any unnatural reductions in anxiety through ritualizing.

ERP treatment has been refined over the years and its use extended to many aspects of OCD. The central principles remain the same, however, and it is worth describing how the approaches were first used, in a case study based on an individual treated some 25 years ago.

John

John had one simple fear – dirt and dirty things. John was not concerned about being infected with any particular disease, and knew that 'dirty things' in themselves were, in the big scheme of things, harmless. However, any contact with dirt made John feel that he was 'dirty', and unless he washed all the dirt away he would feel 'contaminated'. When pressed on what he meant by contaminated, he could not answer, he just said that contamination made him feel tense, disgusted and upset. The only remedy in John's mind was washing until the dirt had gone.

The problem was that washing meant 20, 30 or even more hand-washes, using numerous bars of soap in a week. Sometimes the removal of contamination meant scrubbing with a nailbrush; on his worst days, this entailed John scrubbing himself in the shower until he bled. So, how did exposure and response prevention work?

With John's consent and after a quite lengthy period of discussion, John watched his therapist empty the contents of his waste paper bin onto the floor. The therapist then put his hands inside the waste paper bin, touching all of the surfaces, both inside and out. The therapist then sat there, continuing a conversation with John. John felt very uneasy about the therapist doing this (to say the least), but after his therapy was eventually complete, he mentioned that watching someone else doing something that he would always avoid had helped him somewhat.

This process, of the person with the fear being shown the behaviour that they avoid, is called 'modelling' and years of research have shown that this can be very helpful in the exposure process.

John was then asked to carry out the same actions (emptying the waste paper bin, then touching it inside and out). It became clear that John needed to do this in a very gradual way; thus, the whole process of emptying the bin and touching it inside and out took place over some eight sessions of treatment. The therapist had explained, and agreed with John, the principle that guides exposure – always do what you can just about manage, don't try the impossible. If you do things in small, graduated steps you will get there in the end.

The therapist also demonstrated to John that there was no need to handwash immediately following exposure to the inside and outside of the waste paper bin, and that it was reasonable to wait for a while before washing his hands. The therapist told John that one important issue was to wait until his distress subsided, and that this might take some time. Over the course of treatment, John learned that the distress encountered by emptying the bin and the urges to wash his hands diminished. At first it took 30 minutes for John's distress to begin to subside, but eventually, after several exposures, this reduced to ten minutes or so.

This describes the exposure process in John's case. The second part of ERP, response prevention, was aimed at preventing John from washing his hands on numerous occasions. Once more, the therapist modelled what he considered to be a reasonable hand-wash following the touching of the waste paper bin. Using a modest amount of soap, the therapist took approximately 45 seconds to turn on the taps, put soap on his hands, wash his hands, rinse his hands and then dry his hands with a paper towel. John was asked to copy this behaviour, and although he found it very difficult he managed to wash his hands only once, taking approximately the same time as his therapist.

Following this initial hand-wash, John remained very anxious and upset and wanted to wash his hands again, as he still felt contaminated. John and his therapist talked this through and John was pleased to find that after a few minutes he felt less 'contaminated' and his urges to wash his hands had greatly reduced. When he did wash his hands, if he took longer than the agreed 45 seconds, or reverted to ritualized washing, then this was dealt with by John 're-contaminating' himself by touching the bin and trying again. Thus, the effect of his ritual was 'cancelled out'.

John's sessions of exposure and response prevention were carried out over a number of weeks. Over time, John learned the principles of the treatment and was delighted to find that his distress and his need to hand-wash diminished. After three sessions, John's sister joined the therapy sessions; following some instruction from the therapist, she took over the role of the therapist, demonstrating with the waste paper bin. Eventually, John was able to carry out these exercises alone.

There were other situations that caused John to wash excessively, but the therapy sessions involving the waste paper bin showed a general benefit. Other than the therapist giving some advice about how other situations should be tackled, there was no need to incorporate any of these other situations into therapy sessions.

Many forms of OCD can be tackled with the principle that underpinned John's therapy – for example, the checking of locks and switches. A professional therapist might visit the person's home and demonstrate (model) the appropriate behaviour.

Liz

Liz was a pleasant young woman with an 18-month history of gradually worsening OCD. She had developed obsessional thoughts surrounding something terrible happening to her immediate family (parents, grand-parents, cousins and aunts and uncles). To neutralize these thoughts, Liz had to touch the carpet in her family bathroom with both hands, front and back. Only when she was convinced that she had touched the carpet with every single millimetre of skin would she feel relief and the thoughts would lessen.

At worst, when taking her A-level exams the year before, she was having to ritualize from approximately 7 p.m. every evening until around 2 a.m., and then revise for her exams. Remarkably, and as a reflection of her pure tenacity, she was awarded top marks in all four A-level subjects, and was accepted to study mathematics and physics at Cambridge.

Liz was completely aware that touching the carpet wouldn't really stop anything bad happening, but said that when she had the obsessional thoughts and the anxiety that it caused, it was the only thing that she could do to get rid of them. In addition, she explained that as she was under some stress at the time of her exams, she would think, 'If I do it now, and do it right, then my OCD will leave me alone for a while so I can revise.' So she would do the rituals as a way of trying to stop them occurring later.

Treatment involved explaining to Liz about anxiety and habituation and about the effect that rituals have in terms of only providing short-term relief, but also about them becoming the only strategy that she had. Liz agreed to attempt exposure and response prevention.

Her homework was to sit on her bed, for 40 minutes each morning before breakfast and 40 minutes in the evening, and think about her family members and wait for the thoughts of harm to come. Then she would attempt to stay sitting on the bed and not go to the bathroom to touch the carpet. In the first week of doing this, Liz was able to do it on 10 of the 14 occasions. The remaining four times she 'gave in' and rubbed her hands on the bathroom carpet, which she was somewhat distraught about, saying that she was a failure. Liz was praised, and encouraged to see this as a success, as this meant that she was able to resist the urge to ritualize for over 70 per cent of the exposure time. When she was asked to think about the last time that she was able to resist ritualizing for 70 per cent of a set period of time, in the previous 18 months, she replied that there had never been such a time. Liz was able to see that she was now doing something that she had, up until a couple of weeks ago, been unable to do, and this was an undoubted success.

Liz was then supported to move on in her homework, from exposure to response prevention, as a further strategy. Liz agreed that whenever she ritualized by rubbing her hands on the bathroom carpet, she would imme-diately try and cancel this out by going straight back to her bedroom, taking some photographs of all her 'feared for' family members out of her drawer and imagining that something bad was going to happen to them. This had an excellent effect; the following week, Liz only ritualized once, and immediately did the response prevention task, which she said was 100 per cent successful in cancelling out her ritual and making her anxious again.

After eight sessions, Liz was discharged; at the time of her discharge she had not rubbed her hands against the bathroom carpet for over five weeks. Just as important, she rarely had thoughts of harm befalling her family any more, but realized that if she did, she should allow the thoughts to happen, not ritualize, and let them go away by themselves through habituation.

Iain

Iain was a single 28-year-old who worked in a bank and lived in an apartment complex. He had a seven-year history of OCD related to 'checking' electrical and gas appliances. Over the last year, the problem had significantly worsened and he was finding it almost impossible to leave the house any more, due to the checking rituals that this evoked. He had been signed off sick for four months and his GP referred him for CBT.

Iain explained that although at the time of checking he was 100 per cent sure that the gas and electricity were off, by the time he walked out of the front door of his apartment building, he was instantly hit with the thought, 'Are you sure it is totally off?' He would have further thoughts along the lines of, 'Maybe you accidentally knocked the gas cooker button when walking away without realizing it', or, 'Wasn't that 100 per cent certainty yesterday and not today? Did you even check today?', and so on. Gradually, his doubts would increase and his level of anxiety would slowly rise, until he felt panicky and had to return to check. Iain explained that the gas was his worst fear and the start of his problems, and that while he worried about the electricity, this was less of a concern. His fear was that he would accidentally leave the gas on and cause an explosion in the apartment complex, causing injury and death to his neighbours.

His ritual involved turning the gas tap on, listening for the gas, then smelling the gas, then turning it off and waiting for eight minutes to see if he heard any gas noises or smelt any further gas smells. If he did, then he would repeat the process until he did not. Unfortunately, Iain had also begun developing significant avoidances as a short-term solution. He avoided using the gas at all (for cooking or for central heating) and also had begun to stop using any electrical appliances (apart from light switches). Therefore, he was stuck in his house nearly all day (as to go out would cause massive anxiety), with no gas or electricity.

Treatment focused on using electricity first (as this was the easier of the two fears). Iain agreed to start using some specifically agreed electrical appliances at set times of the day for set time periods. After using them and turning them off, he was to go immediately to his bedroom and resist (fight, even), the urge to go and check that he had turned everything off. After one week, Iain was able to resist checking on 23 of the 35 occasions that he used an electrical appliance. Like Liz, he saw this as a failure, but he was encouraged to view it as a massive success. He had managed to not ritualize on 66 per cent of the occasions he used electricity.

Response prevention was then introduced, and Iain agreed that if he checked the electrical appliance after use, he was to go straight away to his bedroom and tell himself, 'I've left the appliance on, but I'm not going to check', and to visualize the plug smouldering and bubbling as if catching fire, but to not check.

The next week, he reported having completed 31 out of the 35 exposure exercises without ritualizing (a success rate of 89 per cent). Iain was overjoyed at how well he was doing and despite the terrible feelings of anxiety when resisting the need to do his rituals, he noticed that after about 30 minutes he would usually stop feeling anxious, if he 'just stayed with it and did nothing'. Over the course of 12 sessions, Iain was able to tackle all his fears about using electricity and gas and was discharged apart from the occasional follow-up session.

9

Cognitive behavioural therapy

Cognitive behavioural therapy (CBT) is a psychological approach based on scientific principles, which research has shown to be effective for a wide range of problems and clinical conditions. The word 'cognitive' refers to our thoughts and thought processes, and this therapeutic intervention emphasizes the ways in which we think. In CBT people try to identify and understand their problems in terms of the relationship between thoughts, feelings and behaviour, and the effect that these have on mood and day-to-day functioning.

The CBT approach usually focuses on recent difficulties (here and now) you have experienced, and relies on you developing a considered and detailed view of your problems in terms of cognitions and behaviours and how these relate to each other. Based on the understanding of your individual problems, the next steps are to identify goals and develop a treatment plan. The CBT approach is to enable you to generate solutions to your own problems, ways of coping that are more helpful than your present ways, and to test these new ways of thinking or behaving through 'experiments'. This will often involve doing exercises on a daily basis ('homework').

Working with cognitions (thoughts)

An important first step is the process of looking at the evidence concerning our unhelpful thoughts. Unhelpful thinking styles are important because they tend to reflect habitual, repetitive and consistent thought patterns that occur during times of anxiety or depression. As a result, many everyday situations can be misinterpreted. To an extent, these unhelpful thinking styles are a normal part of everyday life, but the fact that they exist means that more helpful (balanced) thoughts are 'crowded out'. We may be more inclined to 'believe' these unhelpful thoughts and not question them, as they reflect how we feel (such as 'down' or 'anxious') and therefore seem to be right.

At one time or another most of us can recognize experiencing at least some of these thinking styles. Usually we can modify and balance this type of thinking. However, during times of greater anxiety or depression unhelpful thinking styles become more frequent, last longer, are more intense, more intrusive, more repetitive and more believable.[8]

Cognitive distortions, or negative automatic thoughts

Cognitive distortions, or negative automatic thoughts (NATs for short), were identified as problems approximately 30 years ago (which was some time after the development of exposure and response prevention). Since that time, strategies to address these distortions have developed, as researchers and therapists observed that some people were unable to complete their ERP therapy. Those people who were unable to tolerate ERP still maintained the attitudes and thinking patterns that prevented them from taking appropriate steps in therapy. For example, in the case of 'contamination', a person might continue to hold the belief that being contaminated is a really harmful thing, although they could not exactly define what harm would befall them. Similarly, someone with sexual or religious obsessions would not take the first step and confront their particular fears, afraid that by doing so they would be guilty of some dreadful sin, or that engaging in their thoughts might cause the person, eventually, to be accused, arrested and imprisoned.

Individuals with these underlying beliefs, thoughts and attitudes would admit, in their less anxious moments, that their fears were illogical and irrational, but would say that at times their beliefs became so strong that they were unable to take any remedial action. It thus became clear that helping some people to modify their thoughts, beliefs and attitudes was necessary. As time has gone on, we have found that during the course of treatment it is helpful to focus on both behaviours and thoughts, and therapists will often discuss underlying thoughts, beliefs and attitudes with those they are treating; in doing so, those with OCD seem to find that their fears are easier to deal with.

Cognitive distortions, or NATs, are those thoughts and ideas that are situation-specific and pop into your mind, causing you to experience some kind of emotional distress. They tend to be very much 'on the surface' and can usually be accessed quite easily in response to questions such as, 'What is going through your mind right now?' or, 'When your mood changed, what were you thinking at that time?' They are common thinking errors that we all make when we are feeling low or anxious; additionally, they tend to be frequent and we tend to 'believe' them.

Table 9.1 lists some of the main thinking errors that people can get trapped into making, with an example of each and how they can be tackled or challenged.

Table 9.1 Thinking errors and how to challenge them

Type of thinking error	Example	What you can do
All or nothing thinking	You see things in black and white, with no middle ground. If your performance falls short of perfect, you see yourself as a total failure.	Think in shades of grey. Try to use words like 'sometimes' instead of 'always', or 'maybe' instead of 'must'.
Fortune-telling	You anticipate that things will turn out badly, your predictions are etched in stone and you feel convinced that your prediction is an already established fact.	Be a detective. Look for the facts. Is there any real or true evidence to back up your prediction? Can you really predict the future?
Jumping to conclusions	You make a negative interpretation even though there are no definite facts that convincingly support your conclusion.	Check things out with others, or in a specific case with the person involved.

Type of thinking error	Example	What you can do
Mind-reading	You arbitrarily conclude that someone is reacting negatively to you, and you don't bother to check this out.	Why jump to conclusions without any real evidence? Actually, what we often imagine is what *we* are thinking about *ourselves*, and we are just fearing that others will take the same view.
Magnification/ catastrophizing	You exaggerate the importance of the situation and predict terrible consequences.	Check the reality of your thoughts – assess the situation by asking questions. What is the evidence that the worst will happen? Has it always happened in the past? A balanced assessment of the risks is always more helpful.
Disqualifying the positive/minimizing	You reject positive outcomes by suggesting that they 'don't matter', or you inappropriately shrink things until they appear tiny (your own desirable qualities or another person's imperfections). This is also called the 'binocular trick'.	Make a list of all that has gone right that day, or ask a friend for their opinion.
Extreme emotional reasoning	You connect the negatives you are feeling with the experience of the situation; for example, 'Because I am nervous, what I have to say must not be important', or, 'I feel it, therefore it must be true.'	Label your emotion and remember that it will pass.

Type of thinking error	Example	What you can do
'Should' statements	You convince yourself to do something with rigid and extreme rules. 'Musts' and 'oughts' are also offenders. The emotional consequences are guilt. When you direct 'should' statements towards others, you feel anger, frustration and resentment.	Eliminate words like 'should' and ask yourself what you would expect someone else to do in the same situation.
Labelling	Mistakes are replaced with labels for yourself that are negative. This is an extreme form of overgeneralization. Instead of describing your error, you attach a negative label to yourself, such as, 'I'm a loser.' When someone else's behaviour rubs you up the wrong way, you attach a negative label to him: 'He's a loser.' Mislabelling involves describing an event with language that is highly coloured and emotionally loaded.	Describe the behaviour or mistake in terms of specific facts and separate the behaviour from your definition of yourself. If you've failed an exam, it means that you've failed an exam – not that you are a failure.
Personalization/ self-blame	You take excessive responsibility for situations that may not even be in your control.	Identify what you could or could not have done about an outcome, then recognize that you did your best. Think of other reasons why people may be saying or doing things. You are not as central in their lives as you think! And be aware of all the people and factors that are responsible for things.

Behavioural changes as a result of thinking errors

In CBT, behaviour is an important factor requiring change; it is often the case that, when we feel different emotions, our behaviour changes as well. The following are some examples.

- Stopping seeing people as often as we once did, thereby allowing thoughts about people not liking us to occur and for such thoughts to be believable. This in turn leads us to see people even more infrequently, and so it goes on.
- Cutting down on socializing, going out, or joining in with others, while experiencing thoughts such as, 'I'm really boring'.
- Taking less interest in hobbies or pastimes, related to thoughts such as, 'What's the point?' or, 'I won't enjoy it'.
- Reducing activities of daily life (such as self-care, housework, or eating), related to thoughts such as, 'I can't do it'.
- Increasing behaviour that attracts attention – sitting staring, or making sudden short movements when feeling angry – which results in others looking at you, causing you to think, 'What are they looking at?'
- Avoiding anxiety triggers (such as shops, when suffering from agoraphobia), leading to a reduction in panic, resulting in thoughts such as 'Avoidance works'.

CBT incorporates behaviours as part of the overall problem, and views the behavioural aspect of experience as both a consequence and a cause of negative automatic thoughts. When you avoid doing things, following thoughts such as, 'I will fail at this', the consequences can be that you end up judging yourself negatively for not doing the things you usually do. You might say, 'I'm a failure', or, 'I can't do anything any more', when thinking about a certain activity. Reduced activity can then maintain your NATs related to anxiety or low mood. As a result, it is unlikely that the veracity of the thought will be challenged. We therefore begin to assume that the thoughts are 'real' or 'true', such as, 'Spiders are dangerous because I get anxious around them.' Avoiding contact with spiders will mean that you will never learn that spiders are less dangerous than you think.

Applying CBT

The thought diary

The cornerstone of the application of CBT is the use of a 'thought diary', as a means of recording your thoughts and emotions and assessing your progress. It can be as basic as an A4 piece of paper. It is a feature of CBT that you use your diary to log the thoughts that are going through your mind (as soon as possible after they have occurred), when you are in the negative emotional state, and then try to find ways of dealing with those negative thoughts, in order to put them in perspective or assess how realistic they are.

The common features of the 'thought diary' include recording the following:

- the date, and the time the problem (or thought) started and ended;
- what you were doing or thinking about when the thought entered your head;
- what emotion the thought evoked (such as shame, anxiety, dread);
- how strong the emotion was, on a 0 to 100 per cent scale, where 0 equals no emotional content whatsoever, and 100 equals the worst you have ever experienced that emotion in your entire life;
- what you tried to do to help deal with the problem situation/ thoughts;
- the outcome – whether what you did actually helped or not;
- how well you think you did in dealing with the problem/thought.

It may be helpful to keep, in addition to the thoughts diary, a 'positive' diary, which contains only achievements and times when you have seen things in a more rational way. Table 9.2 provides an example of a simple thoughts diary.

Table 9.2 Example of a thoughts diary

Situation	Feeling: rate how bad it was (0–100%)	Thought: rate how much you believe this thought (0–100%)	Revised thought: rate how much you believe this thought (0–100%)	Feeling: how bad it was (0–100%)

Socratic questioning

The Greek philosopher Socrates taught his students by asking them questions and drawing out answers. In CBT, we can use Socratic questioning to help uncover the assumptions and evidence that underpin our thoughts in respect of problems. Careful use of these types of questions will enable you to examine your illogical thinking; it is important that your therapist, or anyone helping you with this, maintains an open position that respects the internal logic within even the most seemingly illogical thoughts. Examples of Socratic questions might include:

- Why is that happening?
- How do you know this?
- Show me . . ., or, Prove it.
- Can you give me an example of that?
- What can you learn from this?

Identifying and classifying negative thoughts

In CBT, your thoughts that are associated with OCD are monitored. You may think, 'When I felt low I was thinking that I was going to be alone for ever.' This thought can be classified as a specific type of thinking error (for example, predicting the future). You then ask yourself the following questions: 'If my thought is true, what would that mean to me? Or what would that mean *about* me? Why would that be a problem? What would happen?' For example, if you were rejected or ignored by someone at a party, you may think that you're not attractive. What would happen if you were not attractive? What would happen if you were attractive? How sure of this are you? Could there be another explanation for what happened?

Cost/benefit analysis

It can be often helpful to list all the advantages of having a negative thought, and all the disadvantages.

Examining the evidence

Make a list of the evidence supporting the negative thought, and another of the evidence not supporting the thought. How does the evidence weigh up? What is the quality of the evidence?

Continuum work

You can examine your negative thoughts about specific events based on a continuum, from 0 to 100. Questions to ask yourself might include, 'What will actually happen if the event does occur? What could be worse, better, or the same as a result? What would I still be able to do even if the event does occur?'

Step back and distance yourself from the thought

You may find it helpful to see a particular problem as a thought that you have just had, rather than the actual content of the thought. For example, if you think, 'I am useless', you can change this to, 'I have just had a thought trying to tell me I'm useless.' In essence, you see the thought as the problem, not you.

Imagine your friend . . .

One helpful cognitive technique is to imagine a friend telling you that *they* are experiencing the particular fear or anxiety that you are facing. For example, if you have become obsessed that you may have caused an accident by unwittingly knocking over a cyclist with your car, you might deal with this fear by asking yourself, 'Now, if this was my best friend telling me about this situation, what advice would I give them? Tell them to go back and retrace their journey? Tell them to report the matter to the police, even though there is no evidence of any accident?', and so on.

It is always useful to write down the results of the exercises you undertake. Thus, you not only think about what your friend might say, you have a written record of it.

Take a responsibility holiday

Feeling the need to take responsibility for everything is a characteristic of many people with OCD – for example, ensuring that the house does not get flooded, set fire to or broken into, or, in a public building, worrying excessively about whether the fire exits are impeded, and having to go to check them. One technique that has proved successful is to persuade the person with OCD to take a responsibility holiday.

At home, could you give the responsibility of locking up the house at night to your partner? Either try to go to bed and leave it entirely with them, or you could observe your partner locking the back door, turning on the burglar alarm, and so on. This observation may be helpful because what you will be seeing is 'normal'. If you use this technique, however, try to refrain from commenting on any perceived shortcomings in the process of securing the house!

It is helpful to take responsibility issues situation by situation, perhaps using the example of what your best friend might do if they were in your position, thinking about and writing down how your friend might react in particular circumstances. If you were in a social club, for example, would your friend worry about emergency exits, and go around to the back of the building to ensure that there was nothing blocking the fire doors? Or would they simply say that this was the responsibility of the club manager and leave it at that?

Computerized CBT and self-help

Traditionally, CBT has been delivered by specialist therapists, based either in primary care or in psychological therapy facilities. The limited numbers of therapists compared with the level of demand has led to a situation in which effective psychological treatments are only available to a minority of people who need treatment. The government-funded Improving Access to Psychological Therapies initiative may improve the situation, but for the foreseeable future therapy will reach just a small percentage of those people who need treatment.[9]

Self-help is an alternative to lengthy waiting list delays. It comes in many forms and a range of publications is available.[10] Self-help treatments usually involve written materials (or 'bibliotherapy'), typically providing information about the condition together with instructions on coping strategies, symptom management techniques, self-monitoring, and problem-solving approaches. Over recent years, self-help has also come in other forms, notably computer programs sold over the internet or (for some individuals) available as part of NHS treatment.

NICE recently reviewed their guidance on the use of computerized CBT. It would appear that we still have some way to go before an effective OCD-specific computerized CBT program is developed, but it will probably be only a matter of time. NICE makes the following two recommendations about the use of computerized cognitive behavioural therapy (CCBT) to treat depression and anxiety:

- Beating the Blues, for people with mild and moderate depression
- FearFighter, for people with panic and phobia.

Other programs include COPE and Overcoming Depression for managing depression, but there is currently not enough evidence for NICE to recommend them. They are available for use specifically as part of ongoing or new clinical trials. OCFighter is also not currently recommended for people with OCD, although it is already being used by some as part of a clinical trial.

10

The role of the family

Educating family members about OCD

Family members of those with OCD often feel the need to find out about the nature of the condition; books such as this and many of those listed at the end of this book can be helpful. If you are undergoing professional treatment, your therapist has an obligation to offer advice and answer any questions that your family may have. Although most people with OCD are naturally sensitive about their condition, and there may be aspects of your thinking that you may not wish to share with your family, in our opinion the co-operation and collaboration of the family are essential components of an effective treatment approach. Without education, families often feel that they do not know what to do for the best.

Unhelpful attitudes and behaviours

It is generally true that most families will try to be helpful and aid the individual with OCD. However, sometimes family behaviours can be the opposite, and indeed may make the problem worse. They may be very critical, or sometimes overtly angry, and much of this behaviour may be caused by frustration, because they simply do not understand the obsessional behaviour. Your therapist will need to consider the behaviour of your family, and if necessary try to modify it, usually simply by providing information and education, although alternative approaches may be needed.

Some less than sympathetic families might make fun of the person's behaviour, using the OCD behaviour as a method of embarrassing the individual. While attempting to minimize and prevent such unhelpful behaviour, the use of humour can be a powerful therapeutic tool. The majority of people with obsessional habits will say that they can see the 'funny side' of their behaviour, and therefore some participation in this self-deprecation may actually be helpful. It can provide some levity in the face of anxiety, and demonstrate that the family really do understand. While humour is often used by therapists, however, they do need to get to know you and your family really well before they should attempt to use it as a strategy.

Reassurance-seeking

A very common way in which families try to assist is by verbal reassurance – for example, telling the person that something will not happen, that they will be 'all right'. However, anyone trying to reassure a person with OCD will know that reassurance does not work; but sometimes they do not know what else to do. Therapists often help family members to deal with reassurance-seeking by simple role-playing; instead of providing a reassuring response, they are encouraged to use alternative ways of addressing the request.

Reassurance-seeking in OCD

We all need reassurance from others from time to time – this is normal. Children need normal parental reassurance, as it distinguishes between safe and unsafe, and encourages them in their studies. Adults need reassurance in their working lives, and the appraisal is one tool that is used for this. At a personal level, we seek reassurance from our partners, for instance about how we look; telling your partner that you love them is reassurance-giving, and it is part of the human condition to respond in a positive way to this reassurance.

However, inappropriate or excessive reassurance-seeking is common in OCD, and families often find themselves in a reassurance trap. It is only when they stand back from their situation that they realize that reassurance-giving has become part of the person's problem. Indeed, it serves to make the problem worse.

Questions such as, 'Is this tap off? Is this door locked? Is the car safe? Am I clean? Is this clean? How do I look?' are, on their own, not inappropriate. Within the OCD context, however, particularly given how frequently such questions are asked, they constitute a reassurance-seeking problem. Someone who develops an obsession about an aspect of their health may seek reassurance from their doctor on numerous occasions. There are many examples of people repeatedly seeking testing for HIV, despite the fact that they have never engaged in any risk behaviours.

As mentioned earlier in this book, people of the Roman Catholic faith may go to confession frequently to confess minor transgressions. People with washing and checking rituals may ask others about their cleaning and checking, so that they can give themselves 'extra' reassurance. One woman employed someone to clean her home, specifically the kitchen, bathroom and toilets, in a small three-bedroomed house. She gave her cleaner a very specific list of things to clean and the method of cleaning, and asked her to come in for three hours a day, six days a week. In addition, she spent several hours before and after the cleaner's visit, cleaning the same places. The role of the cleaner was to add to the cleaning that she required. Several cleaners came and went over several months, partly objecting to the fact that they were observed throughout their duties by their employer. She was never satisfied; even after many hours of cleaning, she still felt that her house was 'contaminated'.

Reassurance-seeking often focuses on themes of responsibility. You may seek reassurance that you have not 'done something bad', that you are a 'good person', or that you could not have been responsible for some horrendous event. One man would search local newspapers for reports of indecent exposure; if he found one, he had to ask his wife to reassure him that she knew where he had been at the particular time of the incident.

From the family perspective, reassurance-seeking can damage relationships. Families may find that all conversations centre around aspects of seeking and giving reassurance; normal topics of conversation – the family, weather, politics and so on – are gradually abandoned. Through reassurance-seeking, OCD comes to dominate the lives of both the individual and everyone close to them.

Training families to deal with reassurance-seeking

It is often necessary for therapists to give significant help to family members to deal with excessive reassurance-seeking, using the following steps.

• Information needs to be provided about the role of reassurance-seeking and the maintenance of OCD, and discussed.

- The person with OCD and their family should be encouraged to come to an agreement about what is reasonable.
- A detailed plan of action needs to be set up.

Simply being told not to give reassurance is not adequate. Time needs to be spent with families examining how reassurance-seeking becomes integral to the maintenance of OCD symptoms and how it is detrimental in the long term. Coming to an agreement regarding what is and is not reasonable can also be difficult, and in some cases external advice from a health professional is essential.

When devising a plan, an effective method of dealing with reassurance-seeking is to decide on a simple response to be given on every occasion reassurance is sought, and to ensure that family members do not get drawn into further discussion about the particular topic. For example, one simple response could be, 'I can't answer that question. We have an agreement that reassurance-giving would make the problem worse.'

As part of therapy for OCD, role-play is a technique often used. It can sometimes be helpful to use role reversal – for the person with OCD to take the role of a family member, and the family member to take the OCD role. This may clearly illustrate the damaging nature of reassurance-giving and can be effective in embedding a new response to requests for reassurance.

Family modelling

Many forms of OCD involve behaviours that, simply put, have got out of hand. One of the most common is hand-washing, which may have become very lengthy, systematic and repetitive and a plainly visible abnormal procedure. In order to help the individual, others need to model or demonstrate a reasonable approach. A therapist may wash their hands after touching a waste bin, or the floor, showing what is reasonable, and it will be useful if family members follow suit, so that the individual is able to observe 'normal' behaviour.

However, it is worth repeating a therapist's cautionary tale. In the treatment of an individual with abnormal hand-washing habits, the help of a family member was enlisted as co-therapist. Unfortunately, it was later found that the family member also demonstrated abnormal hand-washing. Sometimes this happens when other members of the family try to adapt to the OCD person's behaviour, and become involved in the ritual. In other cases, it means that other family members have a form of OCD themselves!

11

Looking ahead: relapse prevention

Key questions for those involved in the giving and receiving of treatments for OCD regard their long-term effectiveness – the extent to which the effects of various interventions continue to work following the cessation of treatment – and whether the effects of CBT in particular persist to a greater extent than do those of other treatments.

Evidence suggests that the effects of psychological and especially psychopharmacological interventions substantially weaken, if not disappear entirely, once the treatment is discontinued. However, given CBT's focus on modifying behaviour and thinking and transferring the skills learned in therapy to everyday life, it might be expected that effects would persist, and research studies have demonstrated that gains made during CBT treatment will remain, and a relapse is less likely, once treatment is stopped.[11]

This does not happen without some effort. You will need to practise your weekly targets, and eventually they will become part of your life. This may be more difficult at some times than others – on occasions the obsessional thoughts or urge to act on your compulsions may return or increase in strength, perhaps if your mood becomes depressed or if you experience a serious life event (such as bereavement, or job loss), or have a period of stress.

If you are prone to depression, consider monitoring your mood on a monthly basis. This can be done using a depression questionnaire, for example, the Patient Health Questionnaire 9 (PHQ-9). The PHQ-9 is a nine-item, self-report measure of current depressive symptoms over the preceding two weeks. Scores range from 0 to 27 – the higher the score, the more severe current depressive symptoms. The PHQ-9 can be downloaded free, for clinical use, from <www.depression-primarycare. org/clinicians/toolkits/materials/forms/phq9/>.

It is important to note that OCD does not come back suddenly or immediately. It usually recurs gradually through a series of 'setbacks' – situations where you have difficulty managing obsessional thoughts or a specific situation or trigger causes you to ritualize. A setback is not a relapse. A relapse is when your condition reverts to its original state when it was at its worst. A setback is a time when you need to identify that you are having problems, and work towards dealing with that situation as soon as possible. If you leave it, this will only increase the chance of further setbacks in other areas. If you become depressed, you need to be extra vigilant of the early warning signs of OCD – thoughts or small rituals starting to creep in. Setbacks can usually be nipped in the bud and relapse can often be avoided.

Our advice is that, however you feel, depressed or not, it is useful, particularly for the first year, to monitor yourself to ensure that no thoughts or rituals are beginning. An hour a week could be spent, perhaps on a Sunday, reflecting on your week and honestly appraising whether you have had any difficulties in that time, and coming up with a plan for the forthcoming week if things need to be addressed.

If you have a friend or partner who has helped and supported you through your treatment, it is vital that they are aware of factors that may be associated with a relapse. Ask them to tell you if they notice any rituals beginning, however small.

Conclusion

We hope that this book has met your expectations. Our two central aims were to provide factual information and to set out a programme for self-help. As far as facts are concerned, we are aware that there is a great deal about OCD that is unknown. For example, the mystery remains of how genes and environment interact, or why a certain drug produces excellent results in one person but fails to have much impact on another person with very similar symptoms.

As for self-help, we have drawn on our experience and that of others to develop our advice. It will work for some and not others and there will probably be a need to use a combination of methods. A process of trial and error is required – much the same as with therapy delivered by a professional.

OCD can manifest itself in many ways and its impact on people varies from minor to devastating. We believe that this book, used with or without professional therapy, is a worthwhile tool in the endeavours necessary to deal with this illness, which has such a massive impact, worldwide, on quality of life.

Useful addresses

General

Mind
15–19 Broadway
Stratford
London E15 4BQ
Tel.: 020 8519 2122 (general); 0300 123 3393 (Mind*info*line)
Website: www.mind.org.uk
Helps people to take control over their mental health. There are local Mind groups around the UK.

No Panic
Unit 3
Prospect House
Halesfield 22
Telford
Shropshire TF7 4QX
Tel.: 01952 590005 (office); 0808 808 0545 (helpline)
Website: www.nopanic.org.uk
A voluntary charity, whose aims are to aid the relief and rehabilitation of those people experiencing panic attacks, phobias, obsessive compulsive disorders and other related anxiety disorders.

OCD Action
Suite 506–507, Davina House
137–149 Goswell Road
London EC1V 7ET
Tel.: 020 7253 5272 (office)
Helplines: 0845 390 6232/020 7253 2664
Website: www.ocdaction.org.uk
Provides support and information to anyone affected by OCD, and works both to raise awareness of the disorder among the public and frontline healthcare workers, and to secure a better deal for people with the condition.

OCD Ireland
24 Premier Square
Finglas Road
Dublin 11
Republic of Ireland
Tel.: 01 249 3333 (St Patrick's Hospital Support Helpline)
Website: www.ocdireland.org
A national non-profit support organization for people with OCD, body
dysmorphic disorder and trichotillomania, and their families, friends and
carers. They work through volunteer support groups around Ireland.

OCD-UK
Silverlands Lodge
Boarshead
Crowborough
East Sussex TN6 3HE
Tel.: 0845 120 3778 (office and advice line)
Website: www.ocduk.org

OCD Youth
Young People's OCD Clinic
Maudsley Hospital
Denmark Hill
London SE5 8AZ
Website: www.ocdyouth.info
This site is attached to the clinic for young people with OCD; it publishes a
newsletter, and enables young people to share their experiences of OCD and
to learn how families, friends and teachers can help.

Online resources

Anxiety Care
www.anxietycare.org.uk
A registered charity based in east London; the office in Ilford is now closed
but it continues to operate online with the help of volunteers. It special-
izes in helping people recover from anxiety disorders, and to maintain that
recovery.

Institute of Psychiatry, King's College London
www.kcl.ac.uk/iop/depts/cap/index.aspx
Contains information about obsessive compulsive disorder in children and
adolescents.

International OCD Foundation

www.ocfoundation.org

A non-profit organization based in the United States, it is dedicated to increasing public awareness of obsessive compulsive disorder, as well as providing support and information to those with OCD, their families and friends, and also medical professionals.

National Institute for Health and Clinical Excellence (NICE)

www.nice.org.uk/guidance/index.jsp?action=byID&r=true&o=10975

This section of the website supplies guidelines on obsessive compulsive disorder.

See also: Further reading (NICE).

Oscar Says

www.rachelpiper.me.uk/oscar.html

A person who has experienced OCD provides her story.

Peace of Mind Foundation

www.peaceofmind.com

A website for people who are based in the United States, offering information and support.

Notes

1 <www.nimh.nih.gov/health/topics/obsessive-compulsive-disorder-ocd/index.shtml>.
2 For references in this section, see Anders and Jefferson 1998; Townsley-Stemberger *et al.* 2001; DSM-IV.
3 For references in this section, see WHO 2004; Jenkins *et al.* 1998; Lehtinen and Joukamma 1994.
4 For example, at <www.mysurgerywebsite.co.uk/website/GOSPBC/files/Scales.doc>.
5 See Shin *et al.* 1993.
6 For references in this section, see Department of Health 2001; Newman 2000; Lovell and Richards 2000; Bebbington *et al.* 2000; Marks *et al.* 2003; Abrams *et al.* 1996; Von Korff and Moore 2001; Wilson *et al.* 2000, King *et al.* 2002; Simon *et al.* 2001; Bower and Gilbody 2005.
7 See Bear *et al.* 2007.
8 Williams *et al.* 1997: 72–105, 107–133.
9 See Richards *et al.* 2003, 2009; Department of Health 2008.
10 For example, *Coping with Phobias and Panic* by Kevin Gournay, published by Sheldon Press, 2010.
11 For references in this section, see Hollon *et al.* 2002; Simons *et al.* 1984.

References

Abrams, D., Orleans, C., Niaura, R. *et al.* (1996). 'Integrating individual and public health perspectives for treatment of tobacco dependence under managed health care: a combined stepped care and matching model'. *Annals of Behavioral Medicine*, 18: 290–304.

American Psychiatric Association (2000). *Diagnostic and Statistical Manual of Mental Disorders*, fourth edn (DSM-IV). Arlington, VA, APA.

Anders, J. L. and Jefferson, J. W. (1998). *Trichotillomania: A guide*. Madison, WI, Madison Institute of Medicine.

Azrin, N. H. and Nunn, R. G. (1973). 'Habit-reversal: a method of eliminating nervous habits and tics'. *Behaviour Reversal Therapy*, 11 (4): 619–28.

Barlow, D. H. and Hersen, M. (1984). *Single-case Experimental Designs: Strategies for studying behavior change*, second edn. New York, Pergamon, 1984.

Bear, M. F., Connors, B. W. and Paradiso, M. A. (2007). *Neuroscience: Exploring the brain*. Philadelphia, PA, Lippincott, Williams and Wilkins.

Bebbington, P., Brugha, T., Meltzer, H. *et al.* (2000). 'Neurotic disorders and the receipt of psychiatric treatment'. *Psychological Medicine*, 30: 1369–76 .

Bower, P. and Gilbody, S. (2005). 'Stepped care in psychological therapies: access, effectiveness and efficiency. Narrative literature review'. *British Journal of Psychiatry*, 186: 11–17.

Department of Health (2001). *Treatment Choice in Psychological Therapies and Counselling: Evidence-based clinical practice guideline*. London, Department of Health.

Department of Health (2008). *Improving Access to Psychological Therapies (IAPT) Commissioning Toolkit*. London, Department of Health. May be downloaded from <http://www.dh.gov.uk/prod_consum_dh/groups/dh_digitalassets/@dh/@en/documents/digitalasset/dh_084066.pdf> (accessed 28 June 2011).

Diefenbach, G. J. *et al.* (2000). 'Trichotillomania: A challenge to research and practice'. *Clinical Psychology Review*, 20: 289–308.

Gournay, K., *Coping with Phobias and Panic* (2010). London, Sheldon Press.

Hollon, S. D., Thase, M. E. and Markowitz, J. C. (2002). 'Treatment and prevention of depression'. *Psychological Science in the Public Interest*, 3: 39–77.

Jenkins, R., Bebbington, P., Brugha, T. S., Farrell, M., Lewis, G., Meltzer, H. (1998). 'British Psychiatric Morbidity Survey'. *British Journal of Psychiatry*, 173: 4–7.

King, V., Stoller, K., Hayes, M. *et al.* (2002). 'A multicenter randomized evaluation of methadone medical maintenance'. *Drug and Alcohol Dependence*, 65: 137–48.

Lehtinen, V. and Joukamaa, M. (1994). 'Epidemiology of depression: Prevalence, risk factors and treatment situation'. *Acta Psychiatrica Scandinavica Supplement*, 89(377): 7–10.

Lovell, K. and Richards, D. (2000). 'Multiple Access Points and Levels of Entry (MAPLE): Ensuring choice, accessibility and equity for CBT services'. *Behavioral and Cognitive Psychotherapy*, 28: 379–91.

Marks, I. (1986). *Behavioural Psychotherapy*. Bristol, John Wright. (Now published by I. Marks, London, Institute of Psychiatry.)

Marks, I. M., Maitaix-Cols, D., Kenwright, M. *et al.* (2003). 'Pragmatic evaluation of computer-aided self-help for anxiety and depression'. *British Journal of Psychiatry*, 183: 57–65.

Marks, I. M., Kenwright, M., McDonough, M., Whittaker, M., Mataix-Cols, D. (2004). 'Saving clinicians' time by delegating routine aspects of therapy to a computer: a randomized controlled trial in phobia/panic disorder'. *Psychological Medicine*, 34(1): 9–17.

Merriam-Webster Online Dictionary (2004), www.merriam-webster.com (accessed 21 July 2011).

MSN Encarta Online Dictionary (2010). http://encarta.msn.com (accessed 21 July 2011).

Newman, M. (2000). 'Recommendations for a cost-offset model of psychotherapy allocation using generalized anxiety disorder as an example'. *Journal of Consulting and Clinical Psychology*, 68: 549–55.

NICE, 'Obsessive–compulsive disorder: Core interventions in the treatment of obsessive–compulsive disorder and body dysmorphic disorder'. Clinical Guideline 31 (2005), available from <www.nice.org.uk/cg31> (accessed 21 August 2011).

NICE, 'Computerised cognitive behaviour therapy for depression and anxiety'. Review of Technology Appraisal, 51, available from <www.nice.org.uk/ta97> (accessed 21 August 2011).

Richards, D. A., Lovell, K. and McEvoy, P. (2003). 'Access and effectiveness in psychological therapies: Self-help as a routine health technology'. *Health and Social Care in the Community*,11(2): 175–82.

Richards, D. A., Suckling, R. (2009). 'Improving access to psychological therapies: Phase IV prospective cohort study'. *British Journal of Clinical Psychology*, 48(4): 377–96.

Schulberg, H., Block, M., Madonia, M. *et al.* (1996). 'Treating major depression in primary care practice: eight-month clinical outcomes'. *Archives of General Psychiatry*, 53(10): 913–19.

Shin, J. H., Flaynes, R. B. and Johnston, M. E. (1993). 'Effect of problem-based, self-directed undergraduate education on life-long learning'. *Canadian Medical Association Journal*, 148: 969–76.

Simon, G., Katon, W., Von Korff, M. *et al.* (2001). 'Cost-effectiveness of a collaborative care program for primary care patients with persistent depression'. *American Journal of Psychiatry*, 158: 1638–44.

Simons, A. D., Levine, J. L., Lustman, P. J. and Murphy, G. E. (1984). 'Patient attrition in a comparative outcome study of depression: A follow-up report'. *Journal of Affective Disorders*, 6: 163–73.

Soanes, C. and Stevenson, A. (eds) (2009). *Concise Oxford English Dictionary*, 11th edn. Oxford, Oxford University Press.

Townsley-Stemberger, R. M. *et al.* (2001). 'Personal toll of trichotillomania: Behavioral and interpersonal sequelae'. *Journal of Anxiety Disorders*, 14(1): 97–104.

Von Korff, M. and Moore, J. (2001). 'Stepped care for back pain: activating approaches for primary care'. *Annals of Internal Medicine*, 134: 911–17.

Williams, J. M. G., Watts, F. N., MacLeod, C. *et al.* (1997). *Cognitive Psychology and Emotional Disorders*, 2nd edn. Chichester, John Wiley & Sons.

Wilson, G., Vitousek, K. and Loeb, K. (2000). 'Stepped care treatment for eating disorders'. *Journal of Consulting and Clinical Psychology*, 68: 564–72.

World Health Organization (2004). *The Global Burden of Disease*. See <http://www.who.int/topics/global_burden_of_disease/en/> (accessed 28 June 2011).

Index